The Role of Complementary and Alternative Medicine

Alternative Medicine

Accommodating Pluralism

D0791713

Hastings Center Studies in Ethics

A SERIES EDITED BY

Gregory Kaebnick and Daniel Callahan

This series of books, published by The Hastings Center and Georgetown University Press, examines ethical issues in medicine and the life sciences. Established in 1969, The Hastings Center, located in Garrison, New York, is an independent, nonprofit, and nonpartisan research organization. The work of the Center is mainly carried out through research projects, the publication of the *Hastings Center Report* and *IRB: A Review of Human Subjects Research*, and numerous workshops, conferences, lectures, and consultations. The *Hastings Center Studies in Ethics* series brings the ongoing research of The Hastings Center to a wider audience.

The Role of Complementary and Alternative Medicine

Accommodating Pluralism

Daniel Callahan, Editor

GEORGETOWN UNIVERSITY PRESS / WASHINGTON, D.C.

Georgetown University Press, Washington, D.C. 20007
© 2002 by Georgetown University Press. All rights reserved.
Printed in the United States of America
10 9 8 7 6 5 4 3 2 1   2002
THIS VOLUME IS PRINTED ON ACID-FREE, OFFSET BOOK PAPER.

Permission to rework and reprint some conceptual and textual material for "Personal Experience, Popular Epistemology, and Complementary and Alternative Medicine Resesarch" by Bonnie B. O'Connor was granted by Harwood Academic Publishers, who first published her essay "Conceptions of the Body in Complementary and Alternative Medicine" in Merrijoy Kelner and Beverly Wellman, eds., *Complementary Medicine: Challenge and Change* (Reading, England: Harwood Academic Publishers, 2000).

Support for the writing of "Spirituality in Clinical Care: A Brief Review of Patient Desire, Physician Response, and Research Opportunities" by David B. Larson and Susan S. Larson was provided by Monarch Pharmaceuticals, a wholly-owned subsidiary of King Pharmaceuticals, Inc., Bristol, Tenn., and the John Templeton Foundation, Radnor, Pa.

Library of Congress Cataloging-in-Publication Data

The role of complementary and alternative medicine : accommodating pluralism / Daniel Callahan, editor.
     p. cm. — (Hastings Center studies in ethics)
    Includes bibliographical references and index.
    ISBN 0-87840-877-0 (case : alk. paper)
    1. Alternative medicine. I. Callahan, Daniel, 1930–   II. Series.
R733.R646 2002
615.5—dc21   2001040797

CONTENTS

DANIEL CALLAHAN

Introduction

"Well now, Doctor, just in confidence, I'm going to tell you something
that may strike you as funny, but I believe that foxes' lungs are fine
for asthma, and T.B. too. I told that to a Sioux City pulmonary
specialist one time and he laughed at me—said it wasn't scientific—
and I said to him, 'Hell!' I said, 'scientific!' I said, 'I don't know if
it's the latest fad and wrinkle in science or not,' I said, 'but I get
results, and that's what I'm looking for 's results!' I said. I tell you
a plug G.P. may not have a lot of letters after his name, but he sees
a slew of mysterious things that he can't explain, and I swear I believe
most of these damn' alleged scientists could learn a whale of a lot
from the plain country practitioners, let me tell you!"

Sinclair Lewis, *Arrowsmith*
(New American Library, 1953), 170.

Why did we organize a project on complementary and alternative
medicine (CAM)—a subject not lacking in literature? We did it because
I became curious about an element of the professional debate on the
topic that seemed to me almost inexplicable. How is sense to be made
of the fact that a large and prestigious group of clinicians and biomedical
researchers seems so utterly hostile to CAM while a large portion of
the public (and the educated public at that) seems so attracted to it? Is
it simply a case of the informed squaring off against the ignorant? More
particularly, how is it to be explained that, when the proposal was first
made in the mid-1990s that the National Institutes of Health (NIH)
initiate formal research on CAM, there was such resistance from important parts of the research community? How could researchers, that is,

oppose research on CAM? And, once the NIH had taken on the subject, how could it then fight against any increased budget to do so, even though most other NIH budgets were being increased? Moreover, those opposed to such research seemed—as so often happens with polemics— to harp on only the most egregious examples of bad therapies, bad arguments, and bad actors; that made it easy for them. Was it not possible to find any responsible, thoughtful people sympathetic to CAM? Even more demanding, would it be possible to find people sympathetic to CAM who were also able to approach it with their critical faculties intact and subject it to hard scrutiny?

Those were the questions that sparked this project. Four basic problems needed to be addressed:

- Is there only one acceptable method of scientific evaluation?
- How tolerant should medicine be of different methodologies and standards of evaluation?
- What does it mean to say that a therapy "works" or does not "work"?
- What is a suitable research agenda for alternative and complementary medicine?

While the National Institutes of Health has supported a growing research agenda on complementary and alternative medicine, most of that research has focused on examining the efficacy of various CAM modalities. That is surely important, but there is another issue no less important, hovering in the background. What is the meaning of the public interest? If not just out of ignorance of good scientific methodology, the most convenient explanation, why do so many people turn to CAM? What is lacking in conventional medicine that they seek?

A prominent and long-term science writer for *Time* magazine, Leon Jaroff, suggested that this millennium will bring the end of CAM, wiped out by the superior strength of conventional medical science. This seems most unlikely to me since at least one important attraction of CAM is that it often works at the borderline of those conditions that conventional medicine is not fully capable of managing, most notably chronic conditions. It seems hard to imagine that such borderlines will not always exist, even if they move over the years. It seems no less implausible that conventional medicine will be so decisive in its long struggle with illness, suffering, and death that no one will want anything else. In any event, it is surely possible that the widespread interest in CAM, growing in parallel with conventional scientific medicine as it likewise makes great progress, has something important to say about that latter medicine, if only we know where to look and what to make of what we see.

In putting together a research group to work on CAM, we sought, first of all, those who believe that CAM is a social and medical phenomenon worth taking with full seriousness. Whatever one wants to make of it in the end, it is not something to be dismissed out of hand. Second, we wanted contributors with good critical faculties, aware of the arguments about, and objections to, CAM, but able to make their own judgments. Third, we sought a diverse group with different disciplinary backgrounds. Finally, we wanted a group that could not be subjected to the complaint that CAM is supported by none but the ignorant or self-interested, or that it is opposed to serious efforts to determine efficacy, or that it is just one more way of taking money from the gullible—all charges that can be found in the literature that wants, simply, to get rid of CAM once and for all. All of the contributors to this volume are sympathetic to CAM, take it seriously, and yet are quite willing to subject it to criticism. A number of the contributors, I might add, as well as myself, have never used CAM personally.

The contributors were drawn from medicine, philosophy, research methodology, cultural and folklore studies, and sociology. The chapters fall into two categories: those focused on methodological problems and those focused on cultural perspectives. Yet no sharp line divides the two categories. For just that reason it seemed wise, and perhaps most interesting, to mix the methodological and cultural essays; they reinforce each other in often provocative ways.

Accordingly, the first essay, by Kenneth Schaffner, is written from the perspective of the recent interest in methodological pluralism in the field of philosophy of science. David Hufford is interested in pluralism and diversity as well, but his is a cultural perspective, although one sensitive to the methodological debates. Loretta Kopelman makes a straightforward case that CAM should be judged by exactly the same standards used for conventional medicine. Bonnie O'Connor, however, argues that CAM forces a recognition of the question of whether methodological innovation is necessary for a proper assessment, and argues that the pressure to make sense of CAM pushes strongly in that direction. Howard Brody, focusing on the placebo effect, holds that the gap between CAM and conventional medicine may be much less than most people believe. David Larson and Susan Larson are concerned with assessing the relationship between spirituality and health, reviewing a number of studies to determine the former's impact on the latter. Asbjørn

Hróbjartsson and Stig Brorson take on the difficulty of properly interpreting the results of randomized trials of CAM, upholding rigorous standards. Wayne Jonas takes a broad look at the entire methodological problem of assessing CAM and proposes different levels of assessment. Tom Whitmarsh examines trials of homeopathy and makes the interesting point that physicians using conventional medicine often provide good care for patients despite the absence of randomized clinical trials to validate the treatments they provide. Paul Root Wolpe argues that CAM poses a major challenge to conventional medicine, opening the way to some important changes in the health care system. Alfred Tauber concludes the book with a discussion of all the previous chapters and what he believes the project has achieved. I believe we have achieved a great deal: a better understanding of the dynamic and challenge of CAM and of the relationship between CAM and conventional medicine, and a rich set of suggestions for future research.

We thank the Nathan Cummings Foundation for support of this project.

KENNETH F. SCHAFFNER

Assessments of Efficacy in Biomedicine: The Turn toward Methodological Pluralism

> Before a person studies Zen,
> mountains are mountains and waters are waters;
> after a first glimpse into truth of Zen,
> mountains are no longer mountains and waters are
> not waters; after enlightenment, mountains are
> once again mountains and waters once again waters.
>
> Zen Saying

Once upon a time, all good philosophers of science believed in the unity of science. This included a unity of method for science practitioners. Though they squabbled among themselves whether such unity of method would involve supporting good laws (defended by Dr. Rudolph Carnap) or knocking out big bad theories (pushed by the contrarian Sir Karl Popper), all saw science as true and one. Philosophers even published a book series known far and wide as "The Encyclopedia of Unified Science" with many volumes.

But then a funny thing happened. The last book in "The Encyclopedia of Unified Science" series was *The Structure of Scientific Revolutions* by Tom Kuhn.[1] He said things in science were not as they seemed, and that there were secret rulers he called "paradigms" that could be as different as chalk and cheese. There was no common method! And he had an ally: Paul "The Anarchist" Feyerabend, who preached that unity in science was really bad, and to get science to progress the only rule was no rule, or, as he put it, "anything goes."[2] Then nothing was ever quite the same again.

Science Disunified and Pluralized

This little tale is oversimplified, but it tells of some developments in the philosophy of science and science studies that have current relevance, not only for basic science methodology but also for assessments of complementary and alternative medicine (CAM). Kuhn's and Feyerabend's rich accounts of theories that once looked quite scientific but were subsequently overthrown lent support to what have been termed variously relativist, instrumentalist, or constructivist analyses of scientific theories. Relativists view scientific evidence as relative to an accepted paradigm. Instrumentalists view theories and hypotheses as tools, and not as purportedly true descriptions of the world. Constructivists, such as Latour and Woolgar, conceive of many biomedical entities (e.g., neuroendocrine releasing factors) as being "constructed" rather than "discovered."[3] Similar antiobjectivist themes have been developed by more literary-oriented theorists who take a "deconstructionist" tack.

Such positions as Kuhnian relativism, instrumentalism, and social constructivism are prima facie attractive and even exciting to some, and distressing and outrageous to others. These sociological challenges and the scientists' outrage are all a backdrop to the largely 1990s flirtation of philosophers of science with a methodological pluralism. The methodological approaches range from celebrations of the "disunity" of science,[4] to vigorous defenses of "methodological pluralism,"[5] to a thesis of the "instrumental" nature of most of biology.[6] A good starting point in this area is Dupré's claims about the disunity of science and its methods.

Dupré writes that "no thesis of the unity of science can serve any legitimate purposes for which it might be intended."[7] Further, he writes that, largely due to Kuhn's work, it has become clear that neither is there any *methodological* unity: "there remains no plausibility at all to the prospect of an account of the history of science in which progress is constantly generated by application of a uniform methodology."[8] The centrality of these themes in current philosophy of science is underscored by David Stump. In his section on "Studying the philosophical implications of the unity and disunity of science" in his afterword to a nearly 600-page collection of recent essays on *The Disunity of Science,* Stump writes:

> In accord with the rest of science studies, a central theme of recent philosophy of science has been the view that the methods of science themselves are not unitary. This can be seen in Dudley Shapere's argument that science has developed into independent domains, in the new philoso-

phy of experiment advocated by Ian Hacking and Peter Galison, in which experiment has a life of its own independent of theory, in Arthur Fine's advocating of an antiessentialist view of science as a way of getting beyond debates over realism, in John Dupré's pluralistic metaphysics, and in Thomas Nickles's claim that scientists concern themselves only with domain-specific methods. The disunity of science follows from its contextualization—that is, from studies of the influence of independent domains on the development of science. The disunity of science is crucial to overcoming the realism/relativism debate, and may be our guide in developing a view of science that is radically different from both traditional and relativist views of science.[9]

These disunity views open up the possibility that all methodologies may be local, and that complementary and alternative medicine may be pointing toward methods that diverge legitimately from traditional science. But appeals for a common unified (at least at a general level) methodology have their strong defenders in contemporary medicine.

The Received View: Medicine Does (and Should) Have a Uniform Method

Marcia Angell, M.D., formerly the executive editor of *The New England Journal of Medicine,* articulated the thesis of a uniform method quite clearly in her 1996 book, *Science on Trial.* Dr. Angell wrote:

> Perhaps the most important hallmark of science is its utter reliance on evidence. Furthermore, the evidence must be objectively verifiable. This reliance on concrete evidence distinguishes science from all other human endeavors. . . . Medical conclusions are no different from other scientific matters, because the body is a part of nature. How do medical researchers find the evidence on which their conclusions are based? The approach is quite *uniform*[10] [emphasis mine].

Dr. Angell then sketches this uniform method. It involves asking a question, formulating a hypothesis, designing a study, collecting data, and then analyzing them.

But then the issues begin to get more complex. Actually evaluating medical research, Dr. Angell adds, "is no easy matter" (p. 95). Peer review, often over a period of time and involving different studies, will often be required. Finally, she adds, "We can rarely absolutely prove a hypothesis, although we can gather enough evidence from *enough different studies* to make the hypothesis so probable that we can say it is true for all practical purposes"[11] (emphasis mine).

Some Complications: Types of Studies and Meanings of Evidence

Bracketing the term "enough" in "enough different studies" for a moment, what might we mean by *studies*? It might be worth reflecting for a moment on the diversity of different types of studies that depend on different purposes or different clinical questions. For example, in their article on CAM evaluation in Jonas and Levin's *Essentials of Complementary and Alternative Medicine,* Linde and Jonas list five different kinds of designs typically used to answer five different types of questions.[12] Here I list the question first, with the type of research design in italics after the question:

1. Is the treatment effective for this patient?
   Therapeutic trial with the patient
2. Is the treatment effective on average for patients with conditions like this?
   No-treatment comparison controlled trial
3. Is an aspect of the treatment effective on average for patients with conditions like this?
   Sham- (placebo-) controlled trial
4. For patients with conditions like this, is this a more effective treatment on average than another treatment?
   Two-treatment comparison controlled trial
5. Is the effect biologically demonstrated?
   Laboratory experimentation[13]

These diverse clinical questions are sometimes referred to in the research design literature under the heading of what might be called the three *e*'s: efficacy, effectiveness, and efficiency. In contemporary usage, "efficacy" refers to an intervention that has been shown to be superior to placebo in randomized controlled trials (RCT), or another ideal setting. "Effectiveness" roughly means that the treatment still works when used by the average clinician with the average patient—that is, in the "real world." Finally, and not really raised in the Linde and Jonas questions, the term "efficiency" refers to the level of resources required to produce benefit.

Those terms have different meanings for different writers. Though they seem to date back to Cochrane's work in the early 1970s,[14] Feinstein[15] gives a set of meanings different from Cochrane, and slightly different from those current meanings I just delineated. But I plan not to play the Humpty Dumpty game in this essay, and my meanings agree with the consensus definitions used by the National Information Center on Health Services Research and Health Care Technology (NICHSR).[16]

So, the *studies* we do in a search for evidence are diverse and possibly dependent on the question at hand. But on closer examination, the concept of *evidence* itself becomes complex as well. This complexity is also recognized by evidence-based health workers and in the CAM literature. For example, in a 1999 essay by Spencer we find another list of different types of validation questions dependent on the sense or type of evidence:[17]

Types of Evidence	Validation Questions
Experimental evidence	Is the practice efficacious when examined experimentally?
Clinical (practice) evidence	Is the practice effective when applied clinically?
Safety evidence	Is the practice safe?
Comparative evidence	Is it the best practice for the problem?
Summary evidence	Is the practice known and evaluated?
Rational evidence	Is the practice rational, progressing, and contributing to medical and scientific understanding?
Demand evidence	Do consumers and practitioners want the practice?
Satisfaction evidence	Is it meeting the expectations of patients and practitioners?
Cost evidence	Is the practice inexpensive to operate and cost-effective?
	Is it provided by payers?
Meaning evidence	Is the practice the right one for the individual?

Finally, there is yet another question about evidence that frequently arises in discussions about CAM. This is a question that is probably best framed using the Kuhnian conceptions of paradigm and paradigm shift with which I began my essay. Though it does some injustice to the subtlety of Kuhn's ideas, we can summarize the question in terms of whether evidence is *paradigm dependent*. By this I mean that—from one perhaps overly strident view of the issue—standard notions of diagnostic categories, permissible measurable outcomes, and experimental design criteria represent an imperialistic "Western" mode of thinking that obscures important health results only *evident* from a non-Western perspective. (I should add that some CAM proponents think citing Kuhn and paradigm conflicts and paradigm shifts is detrimental to rational discussion and the *complementary* aspect of CAM.)

Does True Kuhnian Paradigm Conflict Ever Arise in the CAM-COM Relation?

It is important to ask whether a true Kuhnian paradigm conflict ever arises in the relationship between CAM and conventional and orthodox medicine (COM). Though paradigm conflict is often overdiagnosed, and a number of CAM proponents wish to stress the "C" (complementary) and not the "A" (alternative) in CAM, two reasonable examples where we may well find Kuhnian paradigm conflict are available.[18] One involves Ayurvedic medicine, with its strong commitment to cosmic consciousness as the foundation of the universe and its energy-based five elements. A second is traditional Chinese medicine (TCM), which, also in contrast to COM, has a quite different (1) basic set of elements, (2) pathophysiology, (3) differential diagnosis, and (4) set of therapies. I will concentrate on TCM, which is in one form or another more widely known and appreciated in the Western world (it includes acupuncture and Chinese herbal therapy as well as other modalities); this familiarity will allow me to make my points more easily.[19]

TCM's basic set of elements is comprised of two principles (Yin and Yang), five elements (fire, earth, metal, water, and wood), and five bodily components (Qi, or energy, blood, bodily fluids, internal organs, and medians and collaterals [of Qi flow]). TCM's pathophysiology cites three pathogenetic factors: external, internal, and other. Examples of external factors are wind, cold, summer heat, and dampness. Internal pathogenetic factors include seven emotions (joy, anger, melancholy, worry, grief, fear, and fright). "Other" pathogenetic factors include diet, excessive sex, trauma, and parasites. The pathogenetic factors are interpreted with the help of the Yin, Yang, and Qi concepts. Thus, for example, the external factor "wind" is a Yang pathogen, whereas "cold" is a Yin pathogen that tends to impair Yang Qi. Dampness is also a Yin pathogen that can obstruct Qi activities and impair spleen Yang.

There are four diagnostic methods: inspection, a combined auscultation and olfaction, inquiring, and palpation. The information obtained by these methods leads to a differentiation of syndromes (*Bian Zheng*) that are associated with detected abnormalities. TCM has a complex differential diagnosis that can classify medical problems using "eight principles" (yin and yang, exterior and interior, cold and heat, and deficiency and excess). Or the syndrome differentiation can use theories of Qi, blood, and bodily fluids, as well as meridians, among other elements.[20]

Given a probable diagnosis, the practitioner can then consider several different TCM therapeutic approaches. As in its analysis of pathogenesis, the basic elements of Yin, Yang, and Qi figure importantly in restoring appropriate balance in therapy. The TCM practitioner can choose among various principles of treatment, such as controlling the symptom and treating the underlying cause by regulating Yin and Yang and reinforcing antipathogenic Qi. The specifics of treatment principle implementation involve one or more of five modalities: Chinese herbal medicine, acupuncture/moxibustion, Chinese massage and acupressure, mind/body exercise, and Chinese dietary therapy.

These various principles, elements, and methods come together in an illustrative way in a brief case that Lixing Lao reports. He writes:

> A patient with chronic idiopathic nocturnal urticaria was evaluated by an allergist, dermatologist, psychiatrist, and others and was using daily antihistamines, antidepressants, and corticosteroids for several years. No cause for the patient's condition was found. TCM evaluation revealed a *clear energy imbalance [in Qi] along both kidney and lung systems.* Correction of this imbalance with a combination of dietary changes, short-term herbal use, and acupuncture produced elimination of the urticaria, reduction in medication use, and improvement in mood and energy. Had the TCM diagnosis been unclear, this favorable prognosis would not have been expected [emphasis mine].[21]

This case illustrates that the TCM practitioner and her patient may work entirely within the TCM paradigm with respect to both diagnosis and treatment. This short overview of TCM and the instant case thus pose in a pointed way the question of communication and intertranslatability between the CAM and COM worlds. For example, COM has no obvious correlates for Qi, and the elemental chemistry of TCM is not that found in Mendeleev's periodic table.

So, not only do there appear to be different kinds of studies that might be done, and diverse ends to which different studies may be put, but for some the whole framework of experimental study design of COM and its underlying ontologies and methodologies may be foreign to the CAM approach. I am not trying to confuse the reader but am trying to move toward the question of whether there is any general vantage point—think of it as a limited Archimedean point—where we can get some leverage on these complex notions of method and evidence as they have salience in medicine generally and in CAM as well. Further, I want to consider whether such a vantage point might have practical import for physicians, patients, and the many academic medical centers in which CAM is rapidly developing.

"What Works . . ."

We may have the beginnings of such an Archimedean perspective in our concept of an *intervention* and our intuition—that I believe is widely shared—that we can approve of even scientifically suspect interventions, such as homeopathy, *if they work.* The theme of "what works" is one that is quite familiar to CAM debates, and a recent book by Adriane Fugh-Berman, M.D., actually uses that expression as its subtitle.[22]

In trying to come to grips with the complexities of different methods and meanings of evidence and its possible roles in a CAM world, it occurred to me that perhaps this past year's publishing phenomenon might provide some insights. You may know the book *Harry Potter and the Philosopher's Stone,* or a close analogue of it (in the United States it is *Harry Potter and the Sorcerer's Stone*), and its successor books in the series. (Being a philosopher, I have a penchant for the original British title.) I introduce Harry because he is studying to be a wizard at Hogwarts School of Witchcraft and Wizardry, where the core curriculum includes subjects like potions and herbology. Philosophers (there is at least one at Princeton) like to use the notion of an alternative world (or worlds) as a device to clarify issues of interest to this world, and we might do something similar here. We can pose the question: in a world where magic exists, how would Hogwarts Hospital go about deciding how to evaluate in a methodologically sound way what types of therapies (1) to permit their providers to administer, and (2) to endorse as an institution?

Again, I think they would use the idea of "what works." What works at Hogwarts may not work at Harvard (or Mass General) since they are in different worlds. But just as we saw the notion of "evidence" become more complex on analysis, the notion of "works" also has some subtle nuances. Even a simple dictionary definition reveals two dimensions of the notion of *works.* For example, in *The American Heritage Dictionary of the English Language, works* is defined as "to function or operate in the desired or required way." Note there are two senses of (Aristotelian) cause here: (1) efficient cause and (2) final cause (in which a goal state or an evaluated process is assumed and captured by the word *required*). Figure 1 might help to make my points best, where we see as we move down the diagram how the two senses of *works* are divided and how they can be further analyzed.

My thesis is that there are two *core senses* of causation involved in the notion of *works*. The branch on the left in Figure 1 articulates the efficient-cause sense of *works*—as found in our typical concept of causation that we see in common examples such as a baseball breaking a window. That sense can be more deeply analyzed in terms of a manipulation or intervention notion: one intervenes in the world and a change occurs. To block erroneous causal attributions (coincidences), one idealizes the situation and assumes that everything else is held constant, but for the intervention. Since not all interventions are physically possible, it is usual to speak also of the intervention in a "counterfactual" or "hypothetical" way—that is, consider IF the intervention WERE made. . . . . This concept of a manipulation analysis of causation can be made philosophically rigorous; I will not pursue this in the present essay but must refer readers elsewhere.[23] The sense of causation is

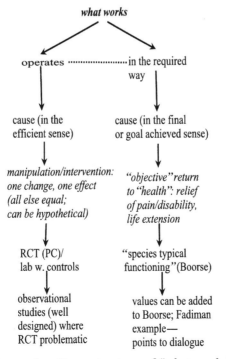

Figure 1. Deep structure of "what works"

also what randomized clinical trials attempt to detect, and what well-controlled laboratory experiments try to divine.[24] Thus I would suggest that Hogwarts Hospital, if they have a research grant review panel as part of their institutional review board, would rank the RCT as the best way to detect evidence that interventions work—whether these interventions are herbal potions or healing spells.

The branch on the right side that elaborates on the phrase "in the required way" identifies a "final" sense of cause inherent in the notion of *works*. I think a core sense of that idea, as understood in the medical area, prima facie points to what is usually referred to as an "objective" notion of health—relief of pain and/or disability and life extension. This notion of an objective account of health has been philosophically defended and deeply analyzed by Christopher Boorse.[25] Boorse's account is controversial but can be taken as a base point for further analyses that can incorporate more divisive cultural notions of health and disease, through a dialogue and negotiation process.[26] Again to return to Hogwarts Hospital, a hospital formulary committee reviewing the evidence for the potion Skele-gro would want to know whether it effectively regrows erroneously removed arm bones to cure that kind of disability.[27]

But reviewing the evidence that tested Skele-gro may be easy compared to the issues raised by the case of nocturnal urticaria discussed above. Hogwarts Hospital committees—and for that matter committees at Mass General as well—would have to have some means of identifying "energy or Qi imbalances" along various systems, or of finding some abnormal correlate discernible in that case. If this is not possible to do in a consistent manner—and here there are different positions that have been voiced[28]—then a less direct means of assessment may be feasible. This less direct evaluation would pool cases of nocturnal urticaria and compare the remedies used (herbal therapy with acupuncture) with placebo and sham acupuncture using an RCT.

But the RCT may itself not be best to detect the effects. The reason for this is indicated in the last part of the branch on the left of Figure 1, which suggests that there can be situations when we need to move beyond RCTs to less rigorous studies. RCTs (including placebo-controlled double-blinded RCTs) may not be feasible or appropriate for a number of reasons. I will not give a detailed catalog of these, but the reader can refer to two recent articles by Black and by Feinstein.[29] Some examples are the presence of obvious effects, the need for a huge sample size or searches for very long-range effects, and interventions that would be unethical.

Black adds another argument against RCTs of special interest to us in the nocturnal urticaria case. He writes:

> Finally, a randomized trial may be inappropriate because the very act of random allocation may reduce the effectiveness of the intervention. This arises when the effectiveness of the intervention depends on the subject's active participation, which, in turn, depends on the subject's beliefs and preferences. As a consequence, the lack of any subsequent difference in outcome between comparison groups may underestimate the benefits of the intervention. . . . The same may be true for many interventions for which clinicians, or patients, or both, have a preference (despite agreeing to random allocation), and where patients need to participate in the intervention—psychotherapy, for example. . . . Many interventions to promote health or prevent disease fall into this category, particularly those based on community development. It is at least as plausible to assume that experimentation reduces the effectiveness of such interventions as to assume, as most researchers have done, that the results of observational studies are wrong. This does not mean there are not scientifically good ways to study such interventions, but a discussion of those would take me beyond my allotted space. Feinstein's article just cited discusses some of these.[30]

Finally, I want to make a general point about diversity of methodology—the topic with which I began this chapter. Within different disciplines some clearly distinct methods are used. Three examples are (1) in molecular genetics, DNA cloning and sequencing of mutations that are tied to their putative effects on the organism; (2) in microbiology, pure culture techniques used to isolate and test by Koch's postulates the putative cause of a disease of the organism; and (3) in neuroscience, nerve stimulation experiments used to test neurotransmitter release at a synapse. These three examples are quite different methods at the fine-structured level regarding techniques, preparations, and instruments. But all seek to determine the effect(s) of a manipulation hypothesized to be the cause of the effect, and all use generally similar methods— what Mill called methods of "difference" (controls) and "concomitant variation" (dose response, quantitative tables of data, and graphs).[31] Example (3) in fact is not even "deterministic" but demonstrates a "probabilistically causal" result (since mini-end-plate-potentials [known as MEPPS] fit a stochastic Poisson distribution).[32]

Thus the disunity of science/method thesis is true, but innocuous, at one fine-structured level, and false, and significantly so, at a more abstract level. Similar points could be made about different types of epidemiological study designs.

Conclusion

The epigraph that began this paper stated:

Before a person studies Zen,
mountains are mountains and waters are waters;
after a first glimpse into truth of Zen,
mountains are no longer mountains and waters are
not waters; after enlightenment, mountains are
once again mountains and waters once again waters.

Before we study CAM we typically subscribe to a standard research design methodology that prioritizes randomized clinical trials and objective measures of health: mountains are mountains and waters are waters. After we study CAM, and think about the arguments of Kuhn and the disunity of science proponents, and about varying local methodologies, we suspect CAM has different evidential standards: mountains are no longer mountains and waters are not waters. But further scrutiny of those arguments and consideration of how CAM practitioners might best go about finding evidence for their claims leads us back to the tried and true methodologies such as RCTs and the need to have agreed-upon measures of abnormal physiology: after enlightenment, mountains are once again mountains and waters once again waters.

But something *has* changed. CAM can help make us realize both that the influence of belief systems may have powerful effects on health and disease and that discerning these effects may require a relaxation of the most Procrustean standards. Alternative belief systems can be examined within other contexts, but this will require tolerance for the alternative claims and complex dialogues as provisional common ground is sought. Those messages seemed to me to have strong support in the papers and discussions that emerged in the course of this project, but those complex dialogues have only begun.

NOTES

1. Thomas S. Kuhn, *The Structure of Scientific Revolutions,* 2d ed. (Chicago: University of Chicago Press, 1970).

2. Paul K. Feyerabend, *Against Method* (London: New Left Books, 1975).

3. Bruno Latour and Stephen Woolgar, *Laboratory Life: The Construction of Scientific Facts* (Princeton, N.J.: Princeton University Press, 1986 [1979]).

4. John Dupré, *The Disorder of Things: Metaphysical Foundations of the Disunity of Science* (Cambridge, Mass.: Harvard University Press, 1993); Nancy Cartwright, *The Dappled World: A Study of the Boundaries of Science* (Cambridge: Cambridge University Press, 1999).

5. Helen Longino, *Science as Knowledge* (Princeton, N.J.: Princeton University Press, 1990).

6. Alexander Rosenberg, *Instrumental Biology or the Disunity of Science* (Chicago: University of Chicago Press, 1994).

7. Dupré, *The Disorder of Things,* p. 221.

8. Dupré, *The Disorder of Things,* p. 233.

9. David Stump, "Afterword," in *The Disunity of Science,* ed. Peter Galison and David Stump (Stanford, Calif.: Stanford University Press, 1996).

10. Marcia Angell, *Science on Trial: The Clash of Medical Evidence and the Law in the Breast Implant Case* (New York: W. W. Norton, 1996), p. 92.

11. Angell, *Science on Trial,* p. 97.

12. Klaus Linde and Wayne B. Jonas, "Evaluating Complementary and Alternative Medicine: The Balance of Rigor and Relevance," in *Essentials of Complementary and Alternative Medicine,* ed. Wayne B. Jonas and Jeffrey S. Levin (Philadelphia: Lippincott, Williams & Wilkins, 1999), pp. 57–71.

13. Linde and Jonas, "Evaluating Complementary and Alternative Medicine," p. 60.

14. A. L. Cochrane, *Effectiveness and Efficiency: Random Reflections on Health Services* (Oxford: Nuffield Provincial Hospitals Trust, 1972).

15. Alvan Feinstein, *Clinical Epidemiology: The Architecture of Clinical Research* (Philadelphia: W. B. Saunders, 1985).

16. See the NICHSR Glossary at http://www.nlm.nih.gov/nichsr/ta101/ta10108.htm; last accessed 21 August 2001.

17. John W. Spencer, "Essential Issues in Complementary/Alternative Medicine" in *Complementary/Alternative Medicine: An Evidence-Based Approach,* ed. J. W. Spencer and Joseph Jacobs (St. Louis: Mosby, 1999), p. 20.

18. I am indebted to Wayne Jonas for suggesting that I look at these two examples.

19. In the following brief account of traditional Chinese medicine, I closely follow Lixing Lao's overview of the subject in his chapter 12, "Traditional Chinese Medicine," in Jonas and Levin, *Essentials of Complementary and Alternative Medicine.*

20. See Lao, "Traditional Chinese Medicine," Table 12.5, p. 223.

21. Lao, "Traditional Chinese Medicine," p. 228.

22. Adriane Fugh-Berman, *Alternative Medicine: What Works* (Baltimore, Md.: Lippincott, Williams & Wilkins, 1997).

23. See the discussion and the references in Kenneth F. Schaffner, "Clinical Trials and Causation: Bayesian Perspectives," *Statistics in Medicine* 12 (August 1993): 1477–94.

24. For further discussion on this topic see chapters 4 and 6 of Kenneth F. Schaffner, *Discovery and Explanation in Biology and Medicine* (Chicago: University of Chicago Press, 1993).

25. Christopher Boorse, "Health as a Theoretical Concept," *Philosophy of Science* 44, no. 4 (1975): 542–73; also see Christopher Boorse, "A Rebuttal on Health," in *What is Disease?* ed. J. Humber and R. Almeder (Totowa, N.J.: Humana Press, 1997), pp. 3–134.

26. I have recently argued that Boorse's account is incomplete but that it can be naturally extended; see Kenneth F. Schaffner, "Coming Home to Hume: A Sociobiological Foundation for a Concept of 'Health' and Morality," *Journal of Medicine and Philosophy* 24, no. 4 (1999): 365–75. For an account of illness freighted with an alternative community's values, see Anne Fadiman, *The Spirit Catches You and You Fall Down: A Hmong Child, Her American Doctors, and the Collision of Two Cultures* (Farrar Straus & Giroux, 1997). For a discussion of how disputes between orthodox and alternative medicine may relate to concepts of health and disease, see B. Lohff et al., "Natural Defenses and Autoprotection: Naturopathy, an Old Concept of Healing in a New Perspective," *Medical Hypotheses* 51, no. 2 (1998): 147–51.

27. J. K. Rowling, *Harry Potter and the Chamber of Secrets* (New York: Scholastic, 1999), pp. 174–75.

28. In a recent presentation, Alvin Feinstein strongly criticized the concept of Qi as nonoperational (Alvin Feinstein, "Evidence-based Medicine and the Assessment of Alternative Medicine," University of Pennsylvania conference on Complementary and Alternative Therapies in the Academic Medical Center: Issues in Ethics and Policy, Philadelphia, November 1999). In remarks from the floor, David Hufford argued that the ability to discern Qi and its imbalances is a skill akin to identifying the differences between good and bad wine vine growths: it can take many years of apprenticeship to learn and it is very difficult to express only in words and measurable quantities.

29. N. Black, "Why We Need Observational Studies to Evaluate the Effectiveness of Health Care," *British Medical Journal* 312, no. 7040 (May 11, 1996): 1215–18; Alvin R. Feinstein, "Problems of Randomized Trials," in *Nonramdomized Comparative Clinical Studies,* ed. U. Abel and A. Koch (Dusseldorf: Symposon Publishing, 1998), pp. 3–13.

30. Black, "Why We Need Observational Studies to Evaluate the Effectiveness of Health Care."

31. For a discussion of Mill's methods and references, see Schaffner, *Discovery and Explanation in Biology and Medicine,* pp. 142–56.

32. This example is discussed in some detail in Schaffner, *Discovery and Explanation in Biology and Medicine,* p. 311.

DAVID J. HUFFORD

CAM and Cultural Diversity: Ethics and Epistemology Converge

Complementary and alternative medicine (CAM) is an aspect of cultural diversity in modern American life, whether found in the ethnomedicine of a newly immigrated group or the widespread CAM utilization of middle-class, Anglo Americans. Ethics and epistemology converge in CAM research because diversity and freedom yield both scientific and social benefits.

In this chapter I will outline and rebut several ideas that have been used to urge sharp limits on diversity in health practice and research. These ideas are common among CAM's most vocal critics, including influential members of the medical establishment. Methodologically, the result of these ideas is preemptive; they do not so much oppose specific methods, but rather pose an obstacle to any kind of research on certain CAM topics. The result is to reduce investigation of widely used practices, the study of which would be likely to raise novel design issues. While arguments about particular design issues are important in the CAM debate, this preemptive bias is even more basic.

I will illustrate these beliefs using recent statements by Dr. Marcia Angell, formerly executive editor of *The New England Journal of Medicine*, but they are not peculiar to her. These beliefs are a common base of opposition to CAM. Many illustrations are conveniently gathered together in *The Scientific Review of Alternative Medicine*, a periodical published by Prometheus Books.

On November 10, 1999, at a conference on CAM held in Philadelphia, Dr. Angell participated in a panel that addressed questions of editorial bias against CAM. Disclaiming bias against good scientific studies of CAM, Angell stated that in order to be good a study must offer a plausible biological mechanism for effects reported. Otherwise, the study would not be believable. She said that therapeutic touch, homeopathy, moxibustion, and intercessory prayer are "preposterous" and "impossible" because they lack a plausible biological mechanism, and that studies of these practices are only being published for social and political reasons. These remarks extended those that she has made in print.[1] Similar comments were made by some of the other editors on the panel.

Dr. Angell is to be complimented for stating this conventional position with great clarity and force. This view hinges on what I will call the theoretical plausibility criterion, in this case the view that the lack of plausible biological mechanisms automatically invalidates the results. Some have attempted to express this criterion in Bayesian terms as prior probability, but prior probability is generally established empirically rather than theoretically and the use of a prior of zero, as Edmond Murphy has pointed out, is an abuse of Bayesian reasoning. In deciding whether a report is accurate or false, a critic using the prior probability argument "evaluates the present evidence *not* (as he should) on its merits but on some multiple of the frequency with which it has previously been reported. . . . If his prior is zero he will never accept any evidence that A occurs."[2]

Plausibility Criteria

"Prior plausibility" is a spurious approach in conventional terrain because it terminates investigation rather than rationally ordering it. The problem is compounded in CAM research, where "the frequency with which the event has previously been reported" is one of the most contested issues. If we are prepared to say that intercessory prayers *have never* produced physical healing or that infinitesimal homeopathic dilutions *have never* produced a biological effect, it will seem reasonable to say that there is no likelihood that they will start doing so now; there is therefore no point in testing the hypothesis that they have these effects. But such effects actually *have* been reported very frequently, and whether these reports are true is part of the issue under investigation. Any claim that belief in the nonoccurrence of such events is empirically founded is circular when accompanied by the assertion that reports of such events should not be investigated. It seems clear that the argument against investigating observations that are "impossible but commonly reported" must be fundamentally theoretical. It rests on confidence that such things *cannot happen* rather than that they *have not* happened. The latter follows from the former, but the distinction is crucial wherever observations are contested.

It should be noted that the interpretation of the alleged observations makes all the difference to whether one believes that *effects* have been observed. After all, no one doubts that people have sometimes recovered following ardent prayer or the administration of an infinitely dilute homeopathic remedy. What is doubted is that the events are causally related, and allegations of *post hoc* reasoning errors are extremely common in the criticism of CAM. But this too may be argued on either empirical or theoretical grounds, and refusal to systematically investigate does not lead to empirical conclusions. For these reasons it is more accurate to discuss this issue in terms of theoretical plausibility than prior probability.

The theoretical plausibility criterion asserts that (1) all valid knowledge will prove to be coherent (that is, to follow logically without inconsistencies or gaps) with some characteristic of established contemporary science (*known biological mechanisms* in Dr. Angell's instance), and (2) that the likelihood that a claim will eventually have this coherent relation to contemporary science can be judged on the basis of present knowledge. Both halves of this assertion are problematic. The assumption of eventual coherence is itself a theory-based prediction that may or may not prove true, and even if it does prove true that does not mean that present knowledge is sufficient to judge which claims may ultimately meet this test.

The theoretical plausibility criterion implies the following, each of which has often been explicitly stated by critics of CAM and all of which are related: (a) Existing conventional scientific knowledge is an adequate measure of whether an unconventional claim is true. Therefore, (b) empirical evidence of an event that is not theoretically plausible can be rejected out of hand. (c) If a practice lacks theoretical plausibility there is no reason to think that it may work. (d) Acceptance of theoretically implausible claims would require the abandonment of current scientific knowledge. (e) There is no such thing as CAM, there is just medicine that is supported by solid research and medicine that is not.

Individually and as a group, these ideas support expert paternalism and suggest that a process of free inquiry open to diverse views is unnecessary and counterproductive in science—except within narrow bounds internal to conventional science. It suggests that the patient's autonomous right to refuse conventional treatment and to use legal alternatives is merely the right to be wrong. This is a view of science as radically transcending cultural and political processes so that the ethical and political mechanisms of a free society are at best a distraction and at worst a destructive force when they intrude on science. This view has profound ethical as well as epistemological implications, and these are especially serious with regard to medical science. My disagreement with the view is not based in a relativizing view of science. Rather it follows from a liberal view of the central importance of free speech in discovering truth and error. I will now provide counterarguments to each of these positions.

The Adequacy of Conventional Scientific Knowledge

Assertions a and b: (a) Existing conventional scientific knowledge is an adequate measure of whether an unconventional claim is true. Therefore, (b) empirical evidence of an event that is not theoretically plausible can be rejected out of hand.

Rebuttal: Dr. Angell's clear and precise articulation of the conventional view is implicitly founded on the kind of reductive unity of science position that was a central part of positivism (both the positivism of Comte and logical positivism), and which Edward O. Wilson has recently championed under the term "consilience."[3] It assumes not only that current knowledge is true, but that all valid future knowledge will be coherent with current knowledge in the strong sense of following logically without inconsistencies or gaps. Such coherence is necessary if all valid knowledge is ultimately reducible to a single set of terms. This idea goes far beyond the reasonable insistence that we should not accept propositions that contradict each other as true. This notion of radical epistemological unity is not widely held in the philosophy of science today.

Even Wilson, while arguing that "the Enlightenment thinkers mostly got it right the first time"[4] and that "[l]ogical positivism was the most valiant concerted effort ever mounted by modern philosophers,"[5] said that this broad view of the unity of valid knowledge "is a metaphysical view, and a minority one at that."[6] Some version of this idea, however, is assumed by many practicing scientists and physicians, and it is often suggested as the only alternative to "relativism." The reductive doctrine assumes a coherent scientific unity of all valid knowledge, present and future, such that new knowledge claims can be evaluated, prior to collecting new data, on the basis of their prospects for assimilation into contemporary science. That which has the potential to be assimilated *may* be true, what does not assimilate *must* be false. This criterion is what Paul Feyerabend calls "the consistency condition," saying it is "unreasonable because it preserves the older theory, not the better theory. . . . It eliminates a theory or a hypothesis not because it disagrees with the facts; it eliminates it because it disagrees with another theory."

He goes on to illustrate with several well-known and entirely conventional examples of the logical inconsistency of accepted physical theories.[7] Dr. Angell illustrated the consistency condition's theory/fact relation as described by Feyerabend when she referred to the moxibustion for breech presentation study published in *JAMA*'s November 11, 1998, alternative medicine issue.[8] The study involved 260 primagravidas in the thirty-third week of gestation, all with breech presentation diagnosed by ultrasound, who were randomly assigned to experimental and control groups. The experimental group received moxibustion, burning moxa rolls over acupoint BL67 (the corner of the fifth toe) seven days in a row, followed by seven more days if the breech presentation persisted. The control group received standard care plus external version if they wished. The study was not blinded.

The moxibustion treatment reportedly produced a rate of cephalic version that strongly favored the experimental group. The results were highly significant in statistical terms ($p = < 0.001$, 95 percent CI) at the thirty-fifth week, and a somewhat smaller, but still very significant, favorable difference at birth. Dr. Angell suggested that since burning *artemisia vulgaris* over the corner of the fifth toe *cannot* affect a fetus, the data showing that it *has* done so must be wrong. In stating this, Angell followed a line common among debunkers. Although he is rarely cited for it, this argument employs David Hume's criterion for when one should refuse to believe a report, described in his 1748 argument against the possibility of a rational belief in miracles: because observation has shown that natural law has never failed, but men have been known to be mistaken or to lie, fraud or error is always a more likely explanation of reports contradicting natural law.[9] Hume said that on hearing such a report there is no obligation to see for yourself, and that if you did see such evidence you should disbelieve your senses (although our senses do not usually lie, sometimes they do, so they too fail as evidence against "natural law").

Dr. Angell supports that conclusion when she says that preposterous studies should not be undertaken or published. But Hume's argument is viciously circular: obviously if one always dismisses conflicting observations, one's beliefs will appear to have a tidy empirical consistency. This circularity is the same as that produced by the abuse of prior probability described above. Because the charge of quackery, meaning medical fraud, is so common in the CAM debate, this rhetorical move is crucial. If novel claims can be attributed to fraud simply because they are novel, despite published, peer-reviewed studies, then scientific objectivity is out the window. Granted, extraordinary claims require extraordinary evidence. But if lack of theoretical plausibility leads to infinitely high standards, good method will be helpless.

The moxibustion theory is not supported by current Western medical theories, but it is supported by the reported facts of the study. It is also supported by the theories of traditional Chinese medicine (TCM). Therefore, Dr. Angell rejects the reported facts rather than questioning the existing theory to which she subscribes. Because the pertinent TCM theories do not make sense within the theoretical framework of Western medicine, they are given no weight. But there is no particular medical theory with which moxibustion or other Qi-based ideas in traditional Chinese medicine disagree. Western scientific theory is silent on Qi, just as it is silent on prayer and the other CAM practices that Dr. Angell finds preposterous. These ideas only conflict with the unity of science doctrine, not with any established scientific knowledge.

Understanding contradiction is central to understanding epistemological debates. That science has no evidence for the existence of Qi does not mean that science has evidence that Qi does not exist. That distinction would be mere sophistry if not for the fact that science has not concerned itself with the investigation of Qi—some scientific evaluation of acupuncture effectiveness, yes, but even the mere existence of Qi, no. Much less does science have evidence that *contradicts* the theory of Qi—that is, firmly supported statements which would be negated by the existence of Qi, its role in health and illness or its manipulation by needling, burning moxa, Qi Gong, etc., such that their conjunction would constitute the statement "p and *not-p*."

Even a strong unity of science view can scarcely propose that observations relevant to all sorts of unconventional or foreign theories have already been made by medical science, as in a claim that "if Qi existed we would have noticed it by now," although such a notion is often implicit in the skeptical reactions of scientists to unconventional claims. When science imagines itself part of a single body of unified truth capable of judging the goodness of other beliefs and practices merely by glancing at them, it is seems to have become somewhat hypertrophied.

Prior to James Reston's 1971 appendectomy in China and the visit to China by President Nixon and his physician Dr. Tkach the following year, all of acupuncture seemed preposterous to most American physicians. Since 1972, empirical inquiry has created a consensus that "something is happening" in Qi-based therapies.[10] That development alone should shatter the canon of prior theoretical plausibility. Western medical science could not have developed acupuncture within the bounds of existing theory. In developing Qi-based therapies Chinese doctors had a great advantage precisely because they did not operate on the basis of modern, Western scientific knowledge. Disbelieving Chinese medical practices on theoretical grounds retarded the development of medical acupuncture and TCM in America for decades and still warps its practice.

The Status of Theoretical Plausibility

Assertion c: If a practice lacks theoretical plausibility, there is no reason to think that it may work.

Rebuttal: This assertion is similar to the dismissal of reports on theoretical grounds, but it goes further. It not only says that such reports must be wrong, but it also implies that those who have reported the observations either do not care that what they report is theoretically implausible in scientific terms (CAM advocates alleged to be hostile or indifferent to science) or do not even know that it is implausible (the general public). For this reason their reports have no weight at all.

Dr. Angell says that it is necessary to have some "reason to believe that a therapy may work" in order to devote resources it. As she put it, rhubarb leaves might help treat cancer—an imaginary example, but not one any less plausible than anything else not yet studied. We cannot study everything at once, so priorities should be based on likelihood of results. Without theoretical plausibility there is no such likelihood. Such skepticism equates the experience of the untrained or differently trained with no reason at all. That is a false equation.

In the 1830s, the popular health reformer Sylvester Graham proclaimed that lack of fiber in the American diet was a great cause of disease. For almost 150 years, generations of reformers repeating this claim, from John Harvey Kellogg to J. I. Rodale to Adelle Davis, were ridiculed by the medical profession for their "preoccupation with bowel movements."[11] Then in the late 1970s when surgeon Denis Burkitt introduced fiber into modern medicine on the basis of several epidemiological and observational studies in Africa, he did not even mention the accumulated observations of thousands in the health food movement.[12] Similarly, beginning in the 1950s the La Leche League advocated for breast-feeding of infants, fighting enormous medical resistance. In 1992, the U.S. Academy of Pediatrics endorsed breast-feeding as superior to formula feeding for American infants,[13] although a national study published in *JAMA* in 1995 showed that despite endorsement of the guidelines many physicians remain ignorant of basic management issues in breast-feeding in ways likely to interfere with the practice.[14]

Such examples could be multiplied manyfold. In each case medicine did not simply remain ignorant of an important health benefit being proclaimed by CAM advocates, but many physicians engaged in practices that unintentionally harmed patients: recommending bland diets and avoiding roughage to patients with digestive problems caused in part by lack of fiber, and employing a variety of obstetric practices that impeded nursing—in some cases even using medication to terminate lactation without the mother's informed consent.

Resistance to health claims coming from outside medicine is generally justified by citing a lack of evidence for those claims. That lack of evidence has the following two sources, among others: refusal to consider accumulated life experience as having any evidential weight, and refusal to turn the attention of medical research to the topic so that conventional scientific evidence could be accumulated. Examples such as fiber and breast-feeding clearly demonstrate that *sometimes* life experience can yield sound knowledge, even when the resulting claims are rejected by legitimate experts in the relevant field. Unlike Qi-based therapies, biological mechanisms for the value of dietary fiber and mother's milk could very easily have been imagined, yet medical researchers showed no interest until many decades after nonscientists had loudly and repeatedly asserted their benefits. That experts dismiss the uncontrolled observations of nonexperts is not hard to explain, no matter how frequently the experts turn out to be wrong. Experts make their livings by producing knowledge that is counterintuitive and that the untrained could not even imagine. It is no surprise that they begin to explain away rather than to listen when confronted with common sense.

In terms of general operating procedures, these examples argue strongly against the idea that theoretical plausibility should be a criterion governing the ability to investigate CAM modalities. Quite the reverse. These examples suggest that many important health findings may well have developed in CAM traditions because those traditions have very different theories that have sponsored very different kinds of observations. And when those health claims are supported by a substantial quantity of experiential reports, those reports should not be dismissed as "mere anecdote" and discounted as evidence supporting a call for inquiry.

It is crucial to add that the presence of a theory or mechanism that conventional theory rejects generally increases the certainty that observations will be rejected. It is not simply that reported effects seem not to make conventional scientific sense, but also that they *do* make sense within some other stigmatized theoretical frame. Graham's theories about physiological overstimulation of the intestines as a source of disease bolstered the rejection of his epidemiological observations, just as TCM theories of Qi and religious beliefs about prayer bolster the rejection of reported effects in acupuncture and intercessory prayer studies. In this, too, theory gains precedence over evidence when unconventional claims meet conventional dogma. If medical research were more open to such outside claims, medical progress would be better served than by a tenacious triumphalism asserting that contemporary medical science already knows everything worth knowing except for those new things which it will discover entirely on its own.

Science and Theoretical Plausibility

Assertion d: Acceptance of theoretically implausible claims would require the abandonment of current scientific knowledge.

Rebuttal: The notion that openness to theoretically implausible claims will demolish science is one of the most frequently heard complaints in the unity of science objection to CAM, and also one of the flimsiest. For example, in 1988 in the editorial accompanying the publication of Jacques Benveniste's in vitro study of homeopathic dilutions in the journal *Nature,* editor John Maddox stated that if Benveniste's findings held up they would require two centuries of scientific progress to be discarded.[15] In the same editorial, Maddox used words such as "supernatural" to describe homeopathic ideas. Such linkages to the spiritual are common in this rhetorical move intended to raise the stakes in the rejection of unconventional claims. While it is silly to call homeopathy supernatural, it is instructive to consider whether even that would justify the claim that science will be stood upon its head and past knowledge abandoned if radical observational claims are honored.

First, the matter of contradiction already noted is central. Do homeopathy or Qi-based therapy and established medical knowledge *contradict* each other? If they did, then accepting one would require rejecting the other. However, they do not. They are simply very different, and their empirical overlap is scant.

To accept the supernatural challenge, we may likewise ask whether medical knowledge is contradicted by intercessory prayer studies, another of Dr. Angell's examples of the preposterous. The randomized controlled trial of prayer in a coronary care unit (CCU) published by Harris and his colleagues in the October 25, 1999, issue of *The Archives of Internal Medicine* provides an apt example. This study tested what is conventionally encountered as a "supernatural belief," namely that prayer can produce divine intervention in illness. But the investigators note of their positive results that "We have not proven that God answers prayer or even that God exists. . . . All we have observed is that when individuals outside the hospital speak (or think) the first names of hospitalized patients with an attitude of prayer, the latter appeared to have a 'better' CCU experience."[16]

Because science is an empirical process, it is hard to imagine a controlled experiment that actually applies to beliefs about God. What was investigated here is a practice that arises from "theories" about God, and the experience of countless millions who believe that they have reason to believe. The study was well crafted in order to investigate something that is readily observable—human behavior and health outcomes. Showing that prayer improves CCU outcomes, if that finding holds up, would not contradict medical knowledge that, for example, lowering cholesterol reduces risk of a myocardial infarction (MI) or that the extent of damage to heart muscle is associated with MI outcomes. The historical decision of science to omit metaphysical issues has been a productive one. But not all religious ideas are entirely metaphysical in the sense of being beyond empirical reach, and if they are not beyond empirical reach, inquiring into them is not antithetical to science.

The claim that ideas foreign to a unified science, especially spiritual ideas, will overturn scientific knowledge is often associated with the claim that those who know science well are not religious in any traditional sense. Dr. Arnold Relman made this statement in his lecture at the Philadelphia conference in November, asserting that science denies religion. This is what distresses advocates of CAM, he says, because CAM, in his view, has a spiritual foundation. He went on to say that, except for a few Deists, there are very few religious scientists.

This idea of religious/scientific incompatibility is inextricable from the view of a unified science with a materialist foundation, from which the demand for a "plausible biological mechanism" arises. It is also an empirical claim, and it is mistaken. Between 1916 and 1996, the level of belief *in a personal God* among American scientists has remained at 40 percent, according to scientific survey data published in *Nature*.[17] This is not the distant God of Deists: the question used in both surveys specified "a God in intellectual and affective communication with human-kind, i.e., a God to whom one may pray in expectation of receiving an answer." The existence or otherwise of God is obviously not something that can be decided by a vote, even a vote among scientists. However, the very high and persistent level of this kind of belief among professional scientists is clear and decisive evidence against the claim that scientific knowledge and religious belief *obviously contradict* one another. Perhaps there is some subtle contradiction. But if so it is not obvious even to scientists, and the burden of proof must be on those who make the claim.

Although the inclusion of spirituality is a common characteristic of CAM approaches,[18] I do not think that most of CAM's theoretical plausibility stands or falls with spiritual belief. However, if even belief in God does not require discarding materialistic scientific knowledge, it seems unlikely that belief in Qi or human energy fields or homeopathic dilutions does. Only contradiction requires that one of two theories be discarded.

Is There More Than One Version of Medicine?

Assertion e: There is no such thing as CAM, there is just medicine that is supported by solid research and medicine that is not.

Rebuttal: If it were true that all valid health knowledge must follow logically without inconsistencies or gaps from conventional scientific theories, then it would follow that, as Wallace Sampson, an energetic debunker of CAM, has said, " 'alternative' and 'complementary' are euphemisms for 'It doesn't work.' "[19] The arguments already offered against the theoretical plausibility criterion also serve against this dis-missal of the entire CAM category, but there are additional, rather more subtle, issues at stake in defining CAM.

In April 1995, the Office of Alternative Medicine of the National Institutes of Health (NIH) held its second conference on research meth-odology. At this meeting I was a member of a working group, chaired by Bonnie O'Connor, that developed the following definition of CAM:

> The broad domain of complementary and alternative medicine (CAM) encompasses all health systems, modalities, and practices other than those

intrinsic to the politically dominant health system of a particular society or culture. CAM includes all practices and ideas self-defined by their users as preventing or treating illness or promoting health and well-being.[20]

This definition is similar to that given by David Eisenberg, who was a member of the working group, and his colleagues in their landmark 1993 study in *The New England Journal of Medicine*,[21] but it broadens the criterion of conventionality beyond theirs of inclusion in medical schools and hospitals. It is intentionally political in scope, and open with regard to conceptual content. It is also neutral with regard to efficacy, and it is not relativistic concerning medical knowledge.

It does not imply that modern conventional medicine has *only* political power to justify its central position. But at all times and in all places there have been powerful social institutions oriented toward health, and there have been other beliefs and approaches that existed in some tension with those institutions. In some places and some times, Western medicine has occupied a CAM role with regard to other healing systems, and in others neither the "politically dominant system" nor its complementary and/or alternative competition was Western.

This definition allows issues such as efficacy and risk-benefit ratios to be addressed as empirical questions worthy of study while also encouraging the investigation of social and cultural issues as intimately related to efficacy claims. The constant criticism to which it has been subjected suggests how important the matter of definition is. Some friendly to CAM have argued that the definition is bad because it marginalizes CAM, defining it by what it is not rather than what it is. In this the definition simply describes the facts: the only thing all CAM approaches share is that they operate outside the margins of the dominant system. There is nothing unusual or necessarily stigmatizing in defining a social fact in terms relative to other social facts: the voters we describe as "Independents" all have in common only that they are not Democrats or Republicans, all suburbs have in common only that they are located outside but near cities, and so forth. In some ways, this relative definition is an advantage in CAM practice today, and in other ways it is a disadvantage. But this is not a weakness in the definition, because the definition was not created to serve a particular ideological goal. The definition was created to provide a useful conceptual tool that would identify the common characteristics among those ideas and practices that are currently referred to when Americans use the words "complementary" and/or "alternative" medicine.

Others, variously disposed toward CAM, have said that the definition is weak because practices that are CAM at one time may be mainstream at another, and because CAM is increasingly taught about in medical schools.[22] The shifting boundaries and changing content of medicine are not weaknesses in the definition, they are also simply a statement of the facts. It is not the job of such a definition to freeze social boundaries, thereby ensuring its own immediate obsolescence. The definition captures the dynamic development of "conventions" within society.

The argument about what is found in medical schools is even less of a difficulty for the definition, but the criticism itself is disingenuous. It is fortunate that in recent years there has been a considerable increase in teaching *about* CAM in American medical schools. When I began teaching on the subject at Penn State's College of Medicine in 1974 I did not know of a single other medical school where such teaching was being done. Today, surveys of the many courses in medical schools are done repeatedly and published frequently. Given the well-established prevalence of CAM utilization by the public, and the possible health implications of that utilization, there are no grounds for arguing that medical students and physicians should remain ignorant of CAM. But most of these courses do not attempt to teach students to *practice* any CAM modality, any more than courses in cultural diversity teach medical students to change their ethnicity. And the extent to which CAM practice itself has penetrated conventional practice is rather small.

But even if CAM were being swallowed whole by conventional medicine, that would not make the definition less accurate. Those who are distressed by the fact that social processes are dynamic and that conventions and institutions change are in for a hard time in the present age of electronic information.

Ethnicity and CAM

This definition should also help to bring greater attention to the place of folk medicine and "ethnomedicine" in CAM. Folk medicine tends to be identified with the cultures of ethnic minorities in the United States, but it is in fact found among all populations.[23] The term usually refers to health traditions that rely heavily on being communicated orally and that are relatively uncommercial. Much folk medicine is community property and does not require a specialist, but specialists do exist within some traditions. Examples of common folk medicine are the association of exposure to cold with predisposing one to getting a cold or other illness, the use of ginger (often ginger ale in the United States) to treat nausea, and beliefs about "hypertension" associating a constellation of conditions with life stress.[24]

The health practices and beliefs of particular ethnic groups are also often called folk medicine, a usage that is sometimes inappropriate— but that is outside the scope of this essay. In addition to folk medicine, the richly varied healing traditions of Native Americans, African Americans, and immigrant communities; the *curanderismo* of Mexican Americans[25] and *brauche* or "powwow" of Pennsylvania Germans;[26] and the pilgrimages to healing shrines practiced by Catholics from diverse ethnic backgrounds[27] all have a strange place in current discussions of CAM. Much of CAM specifically and proudly traces the history of its practices to roots in such traditions, although many in the cultures from which these traditions come consider their appropriation and commercialization by others to be cultural theft. (The misappropriation of Native American religious practice by New Age healers has been especially egregious.) These traditions clearly fit the NIH definition of CAM, they affect health and health behavior, they deserve study, and yet they are rarely brought into explicit discussions of CAM.

The quantitative studies of CAM utilization, from Cassileth et al. in the early 1980s[28] to the 1997 survey by Eisenberg and his colleagues,[29] find CAM utilization much more common among better-educated, white, middle-class Americans than any other group. Although Eisenberg's instrument includes the category "folk remedies," anyone who works with folk medicine will find the very low reported rate of 4.2 percent use within the past year very difficult to believe. It is presumably an artifact of study design. Many factors, possibly including the low response rate encountered by the surveys,[30] and certainly including the restriction of these studies to English-speaking households, has led to the underestimation of CAM prevalence in the nonwhite and non-middle-class population. It is clear that folk medicine and ethnomedicine have been undercounted.

This error has produced a bizarre disconnect in the medical literature. Physicians are urged to be respectfully aware of the "ethnocultural health beliefs and behaviors"—the CAM beliefs and practices—of the least-assimilated members of immigrant groups, assuming that with time these patients will become "more like mainstream patients."[31] At the same time, their colleagues are documenting the widespread use of CAM among "mainstream patients."

The healing traditions of immigrants comprise something that those patients have in common with other American patients. Health culture in the United States is and has always been pluralistic and there are no indications that it is becoming less so. In fact, when Eisenberg and his colleagues published the 1997 replication of their 1990 survey, they found that overall utilization of CAM by the American public had increased from 34 percent to 42 percent. This is part of the cultural diversity of the country. A century of powerful efforts to homogenize American health belief and practice have failed, and they failed for the same reason that the total assimilation associated with the old notion of the American "melting pot" did not occur. Diversity is a natural characteristic of populations, it is adaptive and it can only be suppressed through constant effort. Culturally monolithic societies are like the uniform green lawns of the suburbs or the huge cornfields of factory farms. As soon as the gardener relaxes, wild flowers, trees, and shrubbery return. Whether one deplores or applauds this fact of life, there is no reason today to believe health pluralism will ever go away.

Diversity is represented within the bounds of CAM as well as in the contrast between CAM and conventional medicine. The NIH definition embodies a reminder that in CAM there is no single approach or view, but rather a great variety of views, many having little in common except their medically unconventional nature. The definition also reminds us that this is not a simple grab bag of "remedies" to be considered individually. Throughout modern times intellectuals have made this mistake, assuming that each of the beliefs they do not share, often called superstitions, stands alone. But beliefs do not stand alone. They comprise cognitive systems supported not by single, crucial experiments (any more than medicine is so supported) but by a complex web of reasons within which theory and observation, fact and value, social and cognitive elements intermix.

The existence of shared elements among such systems, even systems that are very different, is to be expected. The isolation of ephedrine from Ephedra Sinica in 1887, and its subsequent introduction into Western medicine by the pharmacological studies of K. K. Chen and C. F. Schmidt, did not remove *ma-huang* from traditional Chinese medicine. Simply because an herbal remedy comes to be used by physicians does not mean that herbalists cease to practice, or that the practice of the one becomes like that of the other. In Ayurveda, gold has been used therapeutically for centuries. In modern times, salts of gold entered

Western medicine. But Western doctors do not use pulse diagnosis in the process leading to the prescription of gold, and salts of gold and gold *bhasma* are prepared in very different ways. The use of acupuncture does not make an American pain clinic into a traditional Chinese medical practice. It is only the assimilationist lens that makes such sharing and mutual influence seem a homogenizing process.

The Cultural Grounding of Western Medicine

The cultural grounding of Western medicine and the existence of CAM modalities within cultural traditions go far to explain contemporary conflicts and interest; they are what make widely used CAM modalities worth investigating. The assimilationist dogma of theoretical plausibility rejects the existence of CAM as a category in order to reduce the issue to a long list of discrete remedies, each of which can and should be tested in the same way and prioritized by standards entirely internal to the traditions of Western medicine. In so doing, it pleads against inquiry into how various and wonderfully diverse configurations of traditions as different as chiropractic and the Navajo Chantway have come into being and thrived. It rejects the idea that health may be defined in a variety of ways or that the context of treatment may make crucial contributions to efficacy quite apart from the hotly debated issue of placebo effect. Part of this criticism of the CAM category has included the assertion that much of what is involved is not *really* medicine but rather lifestyle. This is understandable, seen through the lens of clinical medicine, but that medicocentric assertion should set alarm bells ringing.[32]

The differences in practice between CAM and conventional medicine can be as important as the differences in particular remedies. Compare the practice of a conventional obstetrician to that of a modern midwife providing home birth with medical backup in uncomplicated pregnancies. Numerous studies have shown the safety of midwife-attended home births in women with low-risk pregnancies,[33] and some risks—such as C-section—are even lower for such home births than in hospital births attended by an obstetrician.[34] These midwives have available and use many of the same "remedies" and techniques used by their obstetrician colleagues. But many midwives have a less interventionist approach, greater tolerance for differences in the duration of labor, greater knowledge of and use of the laboring mother's subjective knowledge—a host of differences in style and value that make for a different kind of practice.[35] These differences, when combined with a tendency for midwives to be more interested in botanical medicines, nutritional healing, and the spirituality of childbirth, make some midwives CAM practitioners—even if they sometimes attend hospital births and even occasionally perform episiotomies! Some other midwives are, in contrast, fully integrated within conventional hospital-based obstetric practices.

But this CAM-conventional variation within a health profession should not be a great surprise. For example, a majority of the providers of "alternative cancer treatments" identified in Cassileth's 1984 study were American M.D.s, many with board certification. The penetration of CAM into conventional medicine, and the influence of conventional medicine on all of CAM, from chiropractic to Yoga, has been with us since conventional medicine started to consolidate into recognizable form early in the twentieth century. That interpenetration has never been reducible to the mere integration of specific remedies.

Because the notion of theoretical plausibility has a fundamentally assimilationist thrust, it has given rise to many assumptions about the integration of CAM into conventional medicine. Those assumptions, rather than the political definition, have made CAM seem to be a residual category. The idea that integration of all effective modalities into medicine is the proper goal of CAM research, assumed by many of CAM's most ardent supporters *and* foes, invites the further medicalization of American culture and the co-option and reformulation of CAM modalities. One need only consider the development of medical acupuncture in the United States over the past twenty-five years, whose integration with medicine changed it drastically as it was torn out of its TCM context. The history of osteopathy after the Flexner Report is another poignant example. Many CAM advocates hope to reform medicine through integration, but history suggests that medical co-option will change CAM much more than CAM will change medicine.

Modern medicine does not and cannot do everything that sick people need. Doctors can and should improve their knowledge of the health effects of nonmedical practices, and some CAM practices should be adopted into medical practice, but that does not mean that everything that affects health should be medicalized. It likewise does not mean that, as Congress imagined when setting up the Office of Alternative Medicine at NIH, that "everything that works" should become a part of conventional medicine. That was the idea early in the twentieth century, when medical reform following the Flexner Report aimed to eliminate "sectarian medicine." It did not work then, as the present circumstances amply demonstrate, and it will not work now. Western bio-medicine is a particular tradition of healing that is very good at some of the things that it does and that possesses a body of theory and knowledge that serves it well. But as I have argued elsewhere, both CAM and conventional medicine should be very cautious about integration, even as they struggle toward mutual respect and cooperation.[36] I will reiterate: when scientific medicine imagines itself part of a single body of unified truth capable of judging the goodness of other beliefs and practices merely by glancing at them, it appears to have become hypertrophied.

Process, Not Static Creeds

If the assimilationist dogma of theoretical plausibility were correct, it would follow that the ethical requirement of patient autonomy and the constitutional protections of cultural diversity and free speech conflict with good medical care and productive research. Expert paternalism would consistently trump issues of liberty, at least in matters of epistemology and clinical practice. But the dogma fails on empirical and theoretical grounds. Ethics and epistemology converge in health care as in society at large. There is no medical melting pot because the true unity of science is found in its liberal processes of rational inquiry, not in the allegiance of scientists to a static creed listing beliefs and disbeliefs. The information age is demolishing authoritarian structures worldwide. Isolation has ceased to be an option and domination becomes ever more difficult. Diversity is here to stay, and that means that tolerance of difference has become a practical as well as an ethical necessity. That is true for countries and communities and it is true for intellectual traditions, including Western science.[37] Fortunately, history shows that the confluence of cultures and the process of hybridization increase vigor. Diversity is good in gene pools and good in idea pools too, and for the same reasons.

NOTES

1. Marcia Angell and Jerome P. Kassirer, "Alternative Medicine—The Risks of Untested and Unregulated Remedies," *NEJM* 339, no. 12 (1998): 839–41.

2. Edmond A. Murphy, *Skepsis, Dogma, and Belief: Uses and Abuses in Medicine* (Baltimore: Johns Hopkins University Press, 1981), p. 157.

3. Edward O. Wilson, *Consilience: The Unity of Knowledge* (New York: Alfred A. Knopf, 1998).

4. Wilson, *Consilience,* p. 8.

5. Wilson, *Consilience,* p. 69.

6. Wilson, *Consilience,* p. 9.

7. Paul Feyerabend, *Against Method*, rev. ed. (London: Verso, 1988), pp. 23–24.

8. Francesco Cardini and Huang Weixin, "Moxibustion for Correction of Breech Presentation: A Randomized Controlled Trial," *JAMA* 280, no. 18 (1998): 1580–84.

9. David Hume, "An Enquiry Concerning Human Understanding," Section X, Parts I-II, 1748; reprinted in *Religious Belief and Philosophical Thought*, ed. William P. Alston (New York: Harcourt, Brace & World, 1963), pp. 408–19 .

10. Jane Brody, "U.S. Panel on Acupuncture Calls for Wider Acceptance," *New York Times*, November 6, 1997, p. A10.

11. James C. Whorton, "Patient Heal Thyself: Popular Health Reform Movements as Unorthodox Medicine," in *Other Healers: Unorthodox Medicine in America*, ed. Norman Gevitz (Baltimore: Johns Hopkins University Press, 1988), pp. 52–81, at 74.

12. Denis P. Burkitt, A. R. P. Walker, and N. S. Painter, "Effect of Dietary Fibre on Stools and Transit-Times, and Its Role in the Causation of Disease," *Lancet* 30, no. 2 (1972): 1408–12.

13. American Academy of Pediatrics and American College of Obstetricians and Gynecologists, *Guidelines for Perinatal Care*, 3d ed. (Elk Grove, Ill.: American Academy of Pediatrics; Washington, D.C.: American College of Obstetricians and Gynecologists, 1992).

14. Gary L. Freed et al., "National Assessment of Physicians' Breastfeeding Knowledge, Attitudes, Training, and Experience," *JAMA* 273, no. 6 (1995): 472–76.

15. John Maddox, "When to Believe the Unbelievable," *Nature* 333, no. 6176 (1988): 787.

16. William S. Harris et al., "A Randomized, Controlled Trial of the Effects of Remote, Intercessory Prayer on Outcomes in Patients Admitted to the Coronary Care Unit," *Archives of Internal Medicine* 159, no. 19 (1999): 2273–78.

17. Edward J. Larson and Larry Witham, "Scientists Are Still Keeping the Faith," *Nature* 386, no. 6624 (1997): 436–37.

18. Larry Dossey, *Healing Words: The Power of Prayer and the Practice of Medicine* (New York: Harper Collins, 1993); David J. Hufford and Mariana M. Chilton, "Politics, Spirituality and Environmental Healing," in *The Ecology of Health: Issues and Alternatives*, ed. Jennifer Chesworth (Thousand Oaks,

Calif.: Sage Publications, 1996), pp. 59–71; Robert C. Fuller, *Alternative Medicine and American Religious Life* (New York: Oxford University Press, 1989).

19. David L. Wheeler, "From Homeopathy to Herbal Therapy, Researchers Focus on Alternative Medicine," *Chronicle of Higher Education,* March 27, 1998, pp. A20–A21.

20. Bonnie O'Connor et al., "Defining and Describing Complementary and Alternative Medicine," *Alternative Therapies* 3, no. 2 (1997): 49–57, at 50.

21. David M. Eisenberg et al., "Unconventional Medicine in the United States: Prevalence, Costs, and Patterns of Use," *NEJM* 328, no. 4 (1993): 246–52.

22. Angell and Kassirer, "Alternative Medicine," p. 839.

23. David J. Hufford, "Folk Medicine and Health Culture in Contemporary Society," *Primary Care* 24, no. 4 (1997): 723–41; David J. Hufford, "Folk Medicine in Contemporary America," in *Traditional Medicine Today: A Multidisciplinary Perspective,* ed. Karen Baldwin et al. (Durham, N.C.: Duke University Press, 1991), pp. 14–31; Hufford, "Contemporary Folk Medicine," pp. 228–64; Bonnie Blair O'Connor, *Healing Traditions: Alternative Medicine and the Health Professions* (Philadelphia: University of Pennsylvania Press, 1995).

24. Cecil G. Helman, *Culture, Health and Illness,* 3d ed. (Oxford: Butterworth-Heinemann, 1994).

25. Robert C. Trotter and Juan Antonio Chavira, *Curanderismo: Mexican American Folk Healing* (Athens: University of Georgia Press, 1981).

26. Barbara L. Riemensnyder, *Powwowing in Union County: A Study of Pennsylvania German Folk Medicine in Context* (New York: American Mathematical Society [AMS], 1982).

27. David J. Hufford, "Ste. Anne de Beaupre: Roman Catholic Pilgrimage and Healing," *Western Folklore* 44, no. 3 (1985): 194–207.

28. Barrie R. Cassileth et al., "Contemporary Unorthodox Treatments in Cancer Medicine: A Study of Patients, Treatments, and Practitioners," *Annals of Internal Medicine* 101, no. 1 (1984): 105–12.

29. David M. Eisenberg et al., "Trends in Alternative Medicine Use in the United States, 1990–1997: Results of a Follow-Up National Survey," *JAMA* 280, no. 18 (1998): 1569–75.

30. Eisenberg et al., "Trends in Alternative Medicine Use in the United States," p. 1573.

31. Lee M. Pachter, "Culture and Clinical Care: Folk Illness Beliefs and Behaviors and Their Implications for Health Care Delivery," *JAMA* 271, no. 9 (1994): 690–94.

32. David J. Hufford, "Cultural and Social Perspectives on Alternative Medicine: Background and Assumptions," *Alternative Therapies and Medicine* 1, no. 1 (1995): 53–61.

33. T. A. Wiegers et al., "Outcome of Planned Hospital Births in Low Risk Pregnancies: Prospective Study in Midwifery Practices in the Netherlands," *British Medical Journal* 313, no. 7068 (1996): 1309–13.

34. Carol Sakala, "Midwifery Care and Out-of-Hospital Birth Settings: How Do They Reduce Unnecessary Cesarean Section Births," *Social Science and Medicine* 37, no. 10 (1993): 1233–50.

35. Bonnie B. O'Connor, "The Home Birth Movement in the United States," *Journal of Medicine and Philosophy* 18, no. 2 (1993): 147–74.

36. David J. Hufford, "Integrating Complementary and Alternative Medicine into Conventional Medical Practice," *Alternative Therapies and Medicine* 3, no. 3 (1997): 81–83.

37. Larry Dossey, "'You People': Intolerance and Alternative Medicine," *Alternative Therapies* 5, no. 2 (1999): 12–17, 109–12.

LORETTA M. KOPELMAN

The Role of Science in Assessing Conventional, Complementary, and Alternative Medicines

People around the world spend billions of dollars on food supplements, vitamins, herbal remedies, and traditional therapies. What role should state and federal regulatory agencies have in determining their safety, efficacy, or availability to the public? In passing the Dietary Supplement Health and Education Act of 1994, the U.S. Congress exempted herbals, food supplements, and other complementary and alternative medicines (CAM) from the sort of rigorous testing required for conventional medicines. Defending what it called a "common sense" access to CAM, it places the burden of proof on the Food and Drug Administration (FDA) to show that the product is unsafe.[1] But some people argue that CAM may contain potent agents with powerful adverse effects, and so should be tested as carefully as conventional modalities for safety, efficacy, and standardization as well as their interactions with other drugs. Some countries, such as Germany, do not exempt CAM from rigorous testing,[2] and the United Nations Codex Commission seeks tough worldwide regulatory standards for dietary supplements to be used to guide member countries in developing regulations.

I will argue that CAM should not be exempt from rigorous testing and should be examined using either the best available methods or the same methods used to test conventional therapies.[3] This is because, first, CAM cannot be differentiated well enough from conventional interventions to justify different testing standards. I will argue in the next section that important and well-known proposals about how to separate conventional medicine and CAM fail to distinguish them for the purpose of excusing CAM from rigorous testing standards. If they cannot be clearly distinguished, it is questionable why one set of interventions should be exempt from rigorous testing and another should not.

What constitutes the best available method, of course, will vary with the nature of the intervention, resources, and a variety of theoretical and practical considerations, but labeling something as conventional or CAM does not justify different standards or methods.

Second, I will argue that the same or best available testing methods should be used to evaluate conventional medicine and CAM based on their similarities being held out as therapeutic modalities. This conclusion is based on considerations of (1) the meaning of "therapy" as an intervention intended to be beneficial; (2) duties of therapists, in contrast to quacks and charlatans, to benefit or not harm their patients or clients; and (3) the state's obligations to protect people when they cannot protect themselves or to provide the public good information for prudent consumer choices when they cannot get it themselves. Efficient markets presuppose that consumers have the relevant data to make choices— in this case, about the safety and efficacy of different therapies.

Finally, I argue that while science has a genuine and important role in assessing conventional interventions and CAM for safety and efficacy, this function is limited. In this discussion, the term "therapists" denotes those holding themselves out as providing some form of therapy, whether alternative, complementary, integrative, or conventional.

On Distinguishing Conventional Medicine and CAM

Attempts to distinguish conventional medicine and CAM fall into several groups. Some try to be descriptive and nonjudgmental; others propose normative criteria, saying CAM are untested or fail to meet some scientific standards for rigor adopted in conventional medicine; and still others list specifically what they regard to be CAM. In this section, I argue that these and other attempts fail to distinguish conventional interventions and CAM for the purpose of excusing CAM from rigorous testing standards.[4]

Descriptive: Not in Medical Schools, Hospitals, or the Dominant Health System

The first set of definitions differentiates conventional medicine and CAM descriptively by focusing on what is not taught in medical schools or offered in hospitals. Eisenberg writes: "Alternative Medicine can be defined as medical interventions that are neither taught widely in U.S. medical schools nor generally available in U.S. hospitals."[5]

Eisenberg's definition has been very influential. For example, the American College of Physicians employs a similar definition: "Alternative or complementary medicine is a common term for health practices that are not available from U.S. physicians, are not offered in U.S. hospitals, and are not widely taught in U.S. medical schools."[6] This sort of definition is useful in sensitizing people to the important practices going on outside the walls of medical schools and hospitals and not advocated by dominant health care systems.

Such definitions fail, however, because the standard offered (the fact that something is not taught in medical schools or offered in hospitals or health care systems) is inadequate to distinguish conventional medicine and CAM. First, CAM is getting a great deal of attention in medical schools, hospitals, and by the health care system.[7] Some laws even require that CAM be reimbursed.[8] Second, some medical schools not only teach about CAM, but also have CAM as part of their curriculum.[9] Finally, physiotherapy and some medical subspecialties are part of conventional medicine, yet may not be taught in medical school or offered in some accredited hospitals or by health care plans. Thus, these definitions fail to distinguish conventional medicine from CAM.

Another kind of definition also seeks to be descriptive and nonjudgmental, but characterizes CAM somewhat differently: as health practices outside of the politically dominant health care system. Consider this designation offered by O'Connor and her colleagues:

> Complementary and alternative medicine (CAM) is a broad domain of healing resources that encompasses all health care systems, modalities, and practices and their accompanying theories and beliefs other than those intrinsic to the politically dominant health care of a particular society or culture in a given historic period. CAM includes all such practices and ideas self-defined by their users as preventing or treating illness or promoting health and well-being. Boundaries within CAM and between the CAM domain and the domain of the dominant system are not always sharp or fixed.[10]

This definition usefully acknowledges that conventional medicine and CAM have blurred boundaries, and that what is conventional in one system, culture, or society may be viewed as alternative in others. Herbal teas used for medicinal purposes, for example, may be regarded as CAM in one culture but conventional therapy in another. This proposal also encourages us to reflect on the variety of cultural health practices in the world.

If the goal is to differentiate conventional medicine and CAM in this or other cultures for the purpose of setting different testing standards, however, this definition also has serious problems. It fails to offer a standard for differentiating conventional interventions and CAM other than by appealing to what is or is not intrinsic to the practices of the politically dominant culture. This assumes there is a reliable and useful way to count cultures or subcultures and sort them into those that are dominant and those that are not. A culture is not a nation-state because some social groups have distinctive identities within nations. But if we do not define the dominant culture as the state, how do we distinguish among cultural entities within nations, for example, well enough to say that an action is CAM in one culture but not in another? That is, subcultures in nations typically overlap and have many variations, so how should they be grouped? Even if we could count cultural entities well enough to say exactly how to distinguish one culture from another, how big or old or vital must a culture, subculture, or cult be in order to be recognized as dominant? Even members of the same family may view their drinking of herbal teas or exercise differently; some may do so for pleasure, others as health practices, still others for social purposes, habit, or some combination of reasons. If within the same family some would see these activities as CAM and others not, it would be even more difficult to assess increasingly larger groups. Whose values should we use to count cultures, define what is dominant, or interpret activities as similar enough to be a part of the "dominant culture"?

Defenders might respond that the politically dominant health care culture is comprised of the views of people given authority to run medical schools, hospitals, clinics, or public health departments. Yet they may sharply disagree among themselves and then there would be no dominant view among them. Or, they may disagree with the vast majority of the population about what interventions count as CAM or about their utility. In either case it seems misleading to describe their views as politically dominant, especially if their jobs depend on pleasing the majority. In some countries, for example, ritual burning and female genital cutting are regarded as important health practices by most citizens, yet those running hospitals, clinics, or public health departments in these same countries deplore and try to stop them.[11] Thus, this option fails.

Other defenders might respond that the politically dominant health care culture is the views of the vast majority. One difficulty with this idea is that some of these beliefs are likely to be inconsistent.[12] Since one can formally deduce any statement from a contradiction, this would not be a useful way to distinguish conventional medicine from CAM for the purpose of setting different testing standards. If we amend this proposal by regarding the dominant culture to be whatever is popular with most citizens with the contradictions removed, there is a difficulty of giving a standard for determining which beliefs should be excluded. Thus, this option also fails.

It seems more accurate to describe people as belonging to many overlapping cultures having many variations. Members of the same family may belong to different professional groups or religions, or may marry into families of different racial or ethnic origins.[13] To say we belong to overlapping cultures, however, makes it harder to count cultures or to identify the "dominant culture."

Thus, there can be genuine controversy about whose views represent the dominant culture, with answers depending upon the criteria and values used for distinguishing cultures and dominance. As a result, there are theoretical and practical problems with trying to use this analysis to distinguish conventional medicine and CAM in terms of what is intrinsic to the dominant culture for the purpose of excusing CAM from rigorous testing.

Normative: Untested or Unscientific

Other definitions suggest a standard by which to judge whether some intervention is conventional medicine or CAM based on whether or not the intervention has undergone rigorous testing. The authors of these proposals are generally critical of CAM for their failure to meet these testing norms. Consider the following three quotations. The first is by Angell and Kassier:

> What sets alternative medicine apart, in our view, is that it has not been scientifically tested and its advocates largely deny the need for testing. By testing, we mean the marshalling of rigorous evidence of safety and efficacy, as required by the Food and Drug Administration (FDA). . . . Alternative medicine also distinguishes itself by an ideology that largely ignores biologic mechanisms, often disparages modern medicine science, and relies on what are purported to be ancient practices and natural remedies (which are seen as being somehow simultaneously more potent and less toxic than conventional medicine). . . . [W]ith the increased interest in alternative medicine, we see a reversion to irrational approaches to medical practice, even while scientific medicine is making some of its most dramatic advances.[14]

Barrett says, " 'Alternative medicine' has become the politically correct term for questionable practices formerly labeled quack and fraudulent."[15]

And Sugarman and Burke say, "Conventional modalities (such as surgery and drug therapy) rely on the scientific method whereas alternative medicine modalities (such as acupuncture and therapeutic touch) do not."[16]

These analyses gain credence from studies showing that some CAM are dangerous, untested, or unregulated. Many of the most popular herbals are potent, such as melatonin, ginseng, St. John's wort, and DHEA (dehydroepiandrosterone). In some cases, poor quality control leads to inconsistencies and adulterations with respect to these therapies.[17] CAM can interact with other treatments. For example, PC-SPES is an herbal remedy for prostate cancer, yet it has estrogenic activity. The mixture is often unregulated and may produce clinically significant effects.[18] DHEA is a dietary supplement that increases male and female sex hormones and may cause insulin resistance and hypertension as well as reduce the high-lipoprotein cholesterol. Moreover, only half of the tested products met manufacturer's claims and their variability range was 0 to 15 percent.[19] The use of CAM has also documented dangers to children.[20] There are other examples showing the potent effects of popular CAM and dangers to the public of poor testing and quality control.

Critics are correct that many CAM manufacturers are small-time entrepreneurs who do not test their products and sell small amounts. According to the *Wall Street Journal*, "About 95% of all supplement companies sell less than $20 million in products a year. There are at least a thousand supplement market pushing products, with many upstarts marketing themselves on the Web."[21] The FDA estimates that only about 10 percent of the 22,500 labels that CAM manufacturers are supposed to send to the FDA for review have been sent to them.

Unfortunately, these normative definitions also fail to distinguish conventional modalities from CAM. First, not all conventional treatments advocated within the professional medical community are supported by rigorous testing. The American Academy of Pediatrics concluded that only a small number of drugs and interventions used on both adults and children have had clinical trials performed on pediatric populations; moreover, a majority of drugs on the market have not even been labeled for pediatric populations.[22] The National Institutes of Health (NIH) found that 10 percent to 20 percent of research inappropriately excluded pediatric populations.[23] If poor testing, insufficient information about products, or a lack of will to investigate makes something CAM, as some of these definitions suggest, then, oddly enough, some well-tested interventions for adult populations must be regarded as CAM for children, even if such interventions are used extensively and exclusively in conventional pediatric practice.

Second, some CAM manufacturers adopt higher standards than are currently required in the United States and rigorously test their CAM products. Some even press for higher standards for all manufacturers of CAM so they must use the same standards used for conventional medicine. Thus, conventional medicine and CAM cannot be distinguished solely in terms of whether or not they have been rigorously tested.

Stipulative Definitions

Some definitions simply list what activities they mean by CAM, but unfortunately the lists differ. For example, Astin describes CAM as

> any of the following treatments: acupuncture, homeopathy, herbal therapies, chiropractic, massage therapy, exercise/movement, high-dose megavitamins, spiritual healing, lifestyle diet, relaxation, imagery, energy healing, folk remedies, biofeedback, hypnosis, psychotherapy, and art/music therapy.[24]

Zollman and Vickers give a somewhat different list of common CAM:

> acupressure, acupuncture, Alexander technique, applied kinesiology, anthroposophic medicine, aromatherapy, autogenic, ayurveda, chiropractic, cranial osteopathy, environmental medicine, healing, herbal medicine, homeopathy, hypnosis, mediation, naturopathy, nutritional therapy, osteopathy, Reiki, relaxation and visualization, shiatsu and therapeutic touch, and yoga.[25]

Zollman and Vickers omit exercise and diet, which Eisenberg and colleagues found among the most popular CAM when they conducted telephone interviews. The database Medline also omits diet and exercise under its current classification of "alternative medicine." But Medline includes biofeedback, which Zollman and Vickers omit and Eisenberg and colleagues include. Obviously these and other lists differ. On some lists of CAM, diet, exercise, biofeedback, music therapy, environmental health, art therapy, and nutritional therapy figure prominently. Others omit them, apparently regarding them as conventional modalities.[26]

A related problem is that these stipulative definitions give no justification for excluding some long-standing and popular traditional interventions. As noted, in some regions, ritual burning and/or female genital cutting are regarded as health practices by most citizens.[27] Some reason needs to be given for not including them on the list of CAM.

These stipulative definitions, then, neither successfully distinguish conventional medicine and CAM nor give an account of why some activities should be included as CAM and others not. Until there is substantive agreement about what activities should be included or excluded, stipulative definitions are unlikely to be helpful in distinguishing between conventional medicine and CAM for the purpose of using different testing standards.

Other Proposals

Other suggestions about how to distinguish conventional modalities and CAM are in terms of what is (1) natural, (2) harmless, (3) holistic, (4) unregulated, or (5) not reimbursed.[28] These also fail to offer any basis for distinguishing conventional medicine and CAM in order to set different testing standards. On the first suggestion, the notion of what is or is not natural is very problematic. Many CAM products are processed and have additives so they are not delivered to the consumer in a natural state. Moreover, it is not clear why this feature is relevant since some things in the natural state are deadly poisons. On the second suggestion, what is or is not harmless cannot distinguish them since, as we saw, some CAM are not harmless but are still potent. On the third, many mainstream clinicians are advocates of holistic medicine, so this is not a basis for distinguishing them.[29] Fourth, CAM, especially nutraceuticals, are not unregulated, but may be regulated by less-demanding standards, such as those of good manufacturing practices.[30] For example, CAM must meet such standards in the United States. Moreover, the issue is not what happens to be regulated but what ought to be regulated. As for the final point, some laws require reimbursement of CAM.[31]

In this section, some important and well-known attempts to distinguish conventional medicine and CAM have been explored and rejected as useful for the purpose of excusing CAM from similar testing standards used to evaluate conventional interventions. It is possible that some other definitions or analyses will be able to distinguish between them for this purpose. This seems unlikely, however, since both critics and defenders acknowledge that the boundary between the two is vague and fluid with frequent crossover. Without some way to differentiate them, it is problematic to permit one set of interventions to be exempt from rigorous testing and another not.

Duties to Test Therapies

Conventional medicine and CAM have certain similarities that illuminate the issue of whether they should be evaluated by similar testing standards. In what follows, I argue that three similarities between them offer a basis for a duty to test conventional medicine and CAM for safety and efficacy using the best available or the same methods. The term "therapist" will be used herein to denote all those who intend to provide therapy, including physicians, nurses, and other conventional clinicians, as well as traditional healers and CAM practitioners such as homeopathists, acupuncturists, chiropractors, naturopaths, herbalists, reflexologists, iridologists, macrobioticists, aromatherapists, and electroacupuncturists.

The Meaning of Therapy

One similarity between conventional medicine and CAM is that the interventions are called therapies. To call something a therapy entails both good intentions and some basis for the judgment that it will help people. Therapy, by definition, is something intended to help, not harm, or help more than harm in responding to peoples' pain, suffering, illness, or maladies. The meaning of therapy is linked to this intention, often called *the therapeutic intention*. At one time, people were intentionally infected with the mild viral disease of cowpox to prevent the far more harmful disease of smallpox. People used cowpox as a therapy because the goal was to protect people from a deadly disease. There was a rational basis for that belief because it did provide protection.[32]

While people's good intentions are necessary for something to be a therapy, they are not sufficient to make an intervention a therapy. Many discredited interventions were intended to benefit patients, but their good intentions did not transform them into safe or efficacious modalities. Intentions to benefit do not transform something into an actual therapy. Therapeutic interventions, by virtue of being called therapies, need to in fact help, not harm, or help more than harm patients or clients, creating a duty to test.[33]

Duties of Therapists

What makes someone a therapist is that he or she is competent by some standard adopted by therapists themselves and that he or she honor duties of beneficence and nonmaleficence to those served. People who describe themselves as therapists represent themselves as being able to respond to people's maladies in a way that will help, not harm, or help more than they harm. People trust therapists because they are viewed as having not only certain competencies but also certain duties of beneficence and nonmaleficence. Therefore, people using their knowledge to harm are not therapists. Someone who deliberately infected others with cowpox for no other reason than to make them sick might be providing a therapy (protection against smallpox) in spite of himself, but would not be a therapist because he had no intention of helping the people. If people say a plant is a treatment for cancer but do not believe it, then they deserve to be called quacks, charlatans, or liars, but not therapists. People who deliberately and falsely claim that something will have a therapeutic benefit are lying or deceiving their patients or clients into believing what they do not. Indifference to patients' or clients' safety or unchecked commercial interest should destroy trust in therapists' moral commitments to act in their patients' best interest.[34] For example, if the public learned that surgeons and cardiologists endorse and sell untested or potentially unsafe nutraceuticals, public trust in them and their institutions would probably erode.

At the very least, therapists should believe they benefit their clients. Yet sincerity and good intentions offer no grounds for the belief that therapies are helpful. Justifying the therapeutic intent requires evidence that interventions are safe and efficacious. Thus, when people call themselves "therapists" and their interventions "therapy," they have some duty to justify their claims that the interventions benefit, not harm, or benefit more than they harm. For prudential, economic, as well as moral reasons, therapists want to merit the trust of those they serve. In the case of many CAM, this requires testing.

State Duties to Protect and Supply
Information to Consumers

Another similarity among therapists using conventional interventions and those using CAM is that they generally have some commercial interests, at least by earning income from selling information, services, interventions, or devices. Arguably, the attention that conventional medical institutions are paying to CAM is a result of the large amount of money involved. Eisenberg and colleagues estimate that in 1990, Americans made 425 million visits to CAM practitioners at a cost of over $13 billion.[35] CNN Interactive reports that the amount spent on dietary supplements alone is $13.2 billion in the United States each year.[36] The *Wall Street Journal* estimates the figure at $10 billion.[37]

In business dealings, one ordinarily assumes that competent people can freely fashion their own arrangements for themselves and their dependents and dispose of their fairly obtained property as they wish. The business community assumes that competent people can assess whether or not they want to buy their products, goods, or services, and it believes people should bear the responsibility for their own choices. In contrast, professional relations arise when people cannot assess these things. The economic basis for professions and one of the central reasons patients go to physicians is to obtain good information.[38] Consumers can judge whether and how many bananas, cars, and homes they can afford. They can ordinarily judge for themselves the value of prayer or amulets in their spiritual and physical health. But members of the general public, and most professionals, cannot assess how much surgery they will need in the near future, or the quality of drugs or herbals offered commercially as "therapy." Many of the most popular herbals are potent in themselves or in their interactions with other therapies. These include melatonin, ginseng, St. John's wort, DHEA, and folic acid.[39]

The state has some duty to protect the people when they cannot make assessments for themselves. For example, citizens cannot determine the safety of airplanes, buildings, and bridges on their own, so the state regulates them. It also helps protect them by such means as evaluating the safety and efficacy of conventional treatment modalities and by assessing quality controls and manufacturing practices. People cannot determine on their own what is safe or effective, or when poor quality control leads to inconsistencies and adulterations.

This reasoning can be used to argue that the state also has a duty to assess CAM when people cannot be expected to evaluate whether CAM are safe or effective on their own. That is, this is simply another case where the state has a legitimate duty either to protect people or to give them good information when they cannot get that information on their own. As noted earlier, many of the most popular nutraceuticals have been found potent, unsafe, adulterated, ineffective, or inconsistent. In order for free markets to work in a just society, people need good information. Freedom to choose means little if consumers are manipulated by biased information or cannot get good information in order to make prudent choices. Thus, the inability of the public to assess the safety and efficacy of therapies, whether conventional medicine or CAM, forms a basis for government requirements for safety and efficacy testing. Typically, the government must oversee, regulate, or impose controls so people can be protected when they cannot assess dangers or lack reliable information to evaluate what they purchase.

To summarize, there is no clear way to distinguish CAM from conventional therapies for the purpose of using different testing standards. Their similarities also offer a basis for the duty to test both for safety and for efficacy using the best available or same standards.

The Role of Science

Even if we agree that science should play an essential role in testing conventional medicine and CAM, its role is limited. In some frames of reference, scientific assessments of CAM may even be regarded as incomplete, biased, or irrelevant. Healing rituals within certain religious or spiritual frameworks, for example, may associate physical disease with punishment for bad behavior. Or they may associate therapy with opportunities to repent, become virtuous, or rehabilitate. From a scientific or philosophical aspect, such views may seem implausible. For one thing, it is hard to explain why infants and good people get sick, suffer, and die, while evil people live long and healthy lives.[40] Yet thinking of disease as punishment is an ancient and powerful religious conception. For example, in the Bible, the book of Numbers, chapter 11 verses 31–33, explains the cause of a plague among the Israelites who were finding their way to the promised land:

> Then a wind from the Lord sprang up: it drove quails in from the west, and they were flying all around the camp for a day's journey, three feet above the ground. The people were busy gathering quails all that day, all night, and all the next day and even the man who got the least gathered ten omers. They spread them out to dry all around the camp. But the meat was scarcely between their teeth and they had not so much as bitten it when the Lord's anger broke out against the people and he struck them with a deadly plague.

According to the passage, the plague occurred because the people's disobedience stirred the Lord's anger who struck them with a deadly disease. A scientific framework, in contrast, seeks natural, causal explanations. The quail in the biblical story might have consumed hemlock berries that contained coniine, a neurotoxic alkaloid. Quail are resistant to this poison, but humans are not, so by consuming contaminated quail containing the neurotoxin, they could die. Another natural causal explanation is that the drying period permitted the outgrowth of pathogenic organisms.[41]

One can imagine religious persons, on learning of these scientific explanations or philosophical criticisms of the punishment theory of disease, being no less convinced that God punished the Israelites for being disobedient. Such defenders may believe God sent the quails with their neurotoxic alkaloids or pathogens as a test of the Israelites' faith; they may also accept on faith that if the good die young and the evil live a long and healthy life it fits some divine plan. In this religious framework, explanations and potential cures ignoring disobedience do not get to the essence of the problem. They may seek practitioners with similar views and see scientific explanations as impoverished because the goals, values, and presuppositions of science are so different from those of religion. Scientific explanations or philosophical criticisms will not have the same force in frameworks with different goals, values, and presuppositions about, for example, the role of faith in understanding illness or health.

Despite such limitations, science has an essential role to play in all frames of reference that make causal claims about how to promote health or avoid illnesses. Whether promoting conventional, CAM, or traditional practices, healers asserting their innovations help people make causal claims. Such means-to-ends statements can be justified or refuted even if they are embedded in religious practices. For example, such traditional prevention and healing methods as ritual burning and female genital cutting have been shown to have high morbidity and mortality rates, so they are not a good means to the stated end of promoting health, despite traditional beliefs.[42] In this way, science can support or challenge the empirical claims about how to promote health, cure illnesses, or minimize disabilities, even if they are tied to religious and other cultural beliefs.

Conclusion: The Basis of a Duty to Test

Policies exempting CAM from rigorous testing presuppose some way to distinguish between conventional medicine and CAM. Yet after examining an array of important proposals here, no obvious way was found to clearly distinguish them for the purpose of excusing CAM from testing using the best available or same methods that are used for conventional medicines. Rather, conventional modalities and CAM have some important similarities that serve as a basis for duties to test both using the best available or same methods.

First, a therapy, by definition, is intended to help and not harm, so when therapists present something as a therapy they not only should be sincere, but also have some basis for their claims that something is safe or effective. Second, if therapists hold themselves out as providing therapy, and if a therapy means the therapists intend to help and not harm, then their pledge to help and not harm creates certain duties to use safe or effective therapies. In calling themselves therapists, they say in effect that they can help people. They may intend to help people, but if they know of no justification for their claims, they are being dishonest or deceptive. Third, the state has duties to protect the public when they cannot protect themselves and supply them good information when they cannot get it themselves. For free markets to work, consumers need good information to make prudent choices. The public cannot be expected to know the dangers of some leading CAM currently on the market without such information. For these reasons, CAM and conventional therapies should be subject to the same or best available methods for testing. There is a policy implication of this conclusion, namely that it rejects the reasoning behind the Dietary Supplement Health and Education Act[43] that exempts nutraceuticals from the same rigorous testing required to show the safety and efficacy of conventional drugs.

Although limited, science has a genuine and important role in assessing conventional medicine and CAM by the same or best available methods. Scientific explanations may have a different force in some framework when their goals, values, and presuppositions differ, yet science will at least have an important role in evaluating certain claims, such as in settling disputes over the value of some interventions to fulfill certain goals of health or avoidance of disease. The same or best available methods, therefore, should be used to evaluate the safety and efficacy of both CAM and conventional modalities.

NOTES

1. U.S. Dietary Supplement Health and Education Act of 1994 (DSHEA), Public Law 103-417.

2. Jane E. Brody, "Americans Gamble on Herbs as Medicine," *New York Times*, February 9, 1999, p. F1.

3. I do not discuss what "the same" or "the best available scientific method" may be. In some cases double-blind, randomized clinical trials are best,

in other cases not. Nonetheless, some methods of agreement and difference can be used to make health comparisons among those who do and do not drink herbal tea, exercise, or undergo ritual burning or female genital cutting. Another aspect of this issue is that "the best" method will to some degree depend on the nature of the intervention; for example, potent nutraceuticals would probably require a different and more rigorous examination than amulets.

4. This may not have been their intent since at least some of those offering these analyses would agree that CAM should be tested. Nonetheless, their characterizations are offered as general ways to differentiate them.

5. David Eisenberg, "Advising Patients Who Seek Alternative Medical Therapies," *Annals of Internal Medicine* 127, no. 1 (1997): 61–69; see also David M. Eisenberg et al., "Unconventional Medicine in the United States: Prevalence, Costs, and Patterns of Use," *NEJM* 328 (January 28, 1993): 246–52; David M. Eisenberg et al., "Trends in Alternative Medicine Use in the United States, 1990–1997," *JAMA* 280, no. 18 (1998): 1569–75.

6. American College of Physicians, "Ethics Manual: Fourth Edition," *Annals of Internal Medicine* 128, no. 7 (1998): 576–94, at 581.

7. D. Speigel, P. Stroud, and A. Fyfe, "Complementary Medicine," *Western Journal of Medicine* 168, no. 4 (1998): 241–47.

8. Richard A. Cooper and Sandi J. Stoflet, "Trends in the Education and Practice of Alternative Medicine Clinicians," *Health Affairs* 15, no. 3 (1996): 226–38.

9. Catherine Zollman and Andrew Vickers, "ABC of Complementary Medicine: What Is Complementary Medicine," *British Medical Journal* 319 (September 11, 1999): 8.

10. Bonnie O'Connor et al., "Defining and Describing Comparative and Alternative Medicine," *Alternative Therapies in Health and Medicine* 3, no. 2 (1997): 49–57.

11. Samuel N. Forjuoh, "Pattern of Intentional Burns to Children in Ghana," *Child Abuse and Neglect* 19, no. 7 (1995): 837–41; Loretta M. Kopelman, "Female Circumcision and Genital Mutilation," in *Encyclopedia of Applied Ethics*, vol. 2 (San Diego, Calif.: Academic Press, 1998), pp. 249–59.

12. Examples of such traditional medical practices seem generally ignored in current discussions of CAM, and they are often inconsistent. Arthur Kleinman and Lilas H. Sung, "Why Do Indigenous Practitioners Successfully Heal?" *Social Science and Medicine—Medical Anthropology* 13, no. B1 (1979): 7–26.

13. I argue in more detail in "Female Circumcision and Genital Mutilation" that cultures not only overlap, but some of the views and values within and among cultures seem intertwined with beliefs that are open to rational and empirical evaluation.

14. Marcia Angell and Jerome P. Kassirer, "Alternative Medicine: The Risks of Untested and Unregulated Remedies," *NEJM* 339, no. 12 (1998): 839–41.

15. Barrett goes on to review CAM based upon its having "one or more of the following characteristics: 1. Its rationale or underlying theory has no scientific basis; 2. It has not been demonstrated safe and/or effective by well-designed studies; 3. It is deceptively promoted; or 4. Its practitioners are not qualified to make appropriate diagnoses." Stephen Barrett, "Alternative Medicine: More Hype than Hope," in *Alternative Medicine and Ethics,* ed. James M. Humber and Robert F. Almeder (Totowa, N.J.: Humana Press, 1998), pp. 1–44.

16. Jeremy Sugarman and Larry Burke, "Physicians' Ethical Obligations Regarding Alternative Medicine," *JAMA* 280, no. 18 (1998): 1623–25.

17. For information on the potency of melatonin, see Huijeong Hahm, Jacqueline Kujawa, and Larry Augsburger, "Comparison of Melatonin Products against UPS's Nutritional Supplements Standards and Other Criteria," *Journal of the American Pharmaceutical Association* 39, no. 1 (1999): 27; for ginseng, see "Herbal Roulette," *Consumer Reports* (November 1995): 698; and J. Cui et al., "What Do Commercial Ginseng Preparations Contain?" *Lancet* 344 (July 9, 1994): 134; for St. John's wort see Good Housekeeping Institute, "Consumer Safety Symposium on Dietary Supplements and Herbs," News Release, New York, March 3, 1998; for DHEA, see J. Parasrampuria et al., "Quality Control of Dehydroepiandrosterone Dietary Supplement Products," *JAMA* 280, no. 18 (1998): 1565; Frank LoVecchio, Steve C. Curry, and Teri Bagnasco, "Butyro-lactone-induced Central Nervous System Depression after Ingestion of Renew-Trient, a 'Dietary Supplement.'" *NEJM* 339 (September 17, 1998): 847–48.

18. Robert S. DiPaola et al., "Clinical and Biologic Activity of an Estrogenic Herbal Combination (PC-SPES) in Prostate Cancer," *NEJM* 339 (September 17, 1998): 785–91; Angell and Kassirer, "Alternative Medicine," pp. 839–41.

19. Parasrampuria et al., "Quality Control of Dehydroepiandrosterone Dietary Supplement Products."

20. Max J. Coppes et al., "Alternative Therapies for the Treatment of Childhood Cancer," *NEJM* 339 (September 17, 1998): 846–47.

21. Chris Adams, "Splitting Hairs on Supplement Claims," *Wall Street Journal,* February 22, 2000, pp. B1, B4.

22. American Academy of Pediatrics, Committee on Drugs, "Guidelines for the Ethical Conduct of Studies to Evaluate Drugs and Pediatric Populations," *Pediatrics* 95, no. 2 (1995): 286–94.

23. U.S. National Institutes of Health, "NIH Policy and Guidelines on the Inclusion of Children as Participants in Research Involving Human Subjects," March 6, 1998 [http://grants.nih.gov.grants/guide.notice-files-98-024.html].

24. John Astin, "Why Patients Use Alternative Medicine: Results of a National Study," *JAMA* 279, no. 19 (1998): 1548–53.

25. Zollman and Vickers, "ABC of Complementary Medicine," p. 8.

26. At a recent meeting of many of the authors of this volume, someone asked how many people present use CAM. A long discussion followed about what the person thought CAM meant before we could vote. The person did not, for example, think that exercise should be included as CAM, even though, as noted, Eisenberg and colleagues found the public regarded it as one of the most popular forms of CAM. Eisenberg et al., "Trends in Alternative Medicine Use in the United States."

27. Forjuoh, "Pattern of Intentional Burns to Children in Ghana," pp. 837–41; Kopelman, "Female Circumcision and Genital Mutilation," pp. 249–59.

28. Zollman and Vickers, "ABC of Complementary Medicine."

29. Loretta M. Kopelman and John Moskop, "The Holistic Health Movement: A Survey and Critique," *Journal of Medicine and Philosophy* 6 (May 1981): 209–35.

30. Brody, "Americans Gamble on Herbs as Medicine," p. 1.

31. Cooper and Stoflet, "Trends in the Education and Practice of Alternative Medicine Clinicians," pp. 226–38.

32. According to Ernst, therapeutic opinions by CAM practitioners are more likely to be based on opinion than evidence. Edzard Ernst, "The Ethics of Complementary Medicine," *Journal of Medical Ethics* 22 (1996): 97–198.

33. A related point is that the Food and Drug Administration (FDA) recently attempted to hold that some CAM claims must go through the FDA despite the DSHEA exemptions. The FDA argues that testing must back up claims that CAM interventions improve the structure or function of the body or help fight a disease (Adams, "Splitting Hairs on Supplement Claims"). This criticism would not apply to self-medicators.

34. Edmund D. Pellegrino and Arnold S. Relman, "Professional Medical Associations: Ethical and Practical Guidelines," *JAMA* 282, no. 10 (1999): 984–86; Loretta M. Kopelman and Michael G. Palumbo, "The U.S. Health Delivery System: Inefficient and Unfair to Children," *American Journal of Law and Medicine* 23, no. 2–3 (1997): 319–37.

35. Eisenberg, "Advising Patients Who Seek Alternative Medical Therapies," pp. 61–69; Eisenberg et al., "Trends in Alternative Medicine Use in the United States," pp. 1569–75; also see Astin, "Why Patients Use Alternative Medicine," pp. 1548–53.

36. CNN Interactive, February 22, 1998 [http://europe.cnn.com/HEALTH/9802/22/supplement.safety].

37. Adams, "Splitting Hairs on Supplement Claims," pp. B1, B4.

38. Kopelman and Palumbo, "The U.S. Health Delivery System," pp. 319–37.

39. Hahm, "Comparison of Melatonin Products," p. 27; "Herbal Roulette," p. 698; Cui et al., "What Do Commercial Ginseng Preparations Contain?" p. 134; Good Housekeeping Institute, "Consumer Safety Symposium on Dietary Supplements and Herbs"; Parasrampuria et al., "Quality Control of Dehydroepiandrosterone Dietary Supplement Products"; S. W. Hoag, H. Ramachandroni, and R. F. Shangraw, "The Failure of Prescription Prenatal Vitamin Products to Meet USP Standards for Folic Acid Dissolution," *Journal of the American Pharmaceutical Association* 4 (July 1999): 397–400.

40. Loretta M. Kopelman, "The Punishment Concept of Disease," in *AIDS: Ethics and Public Policy,* ed. Christine Pierce and Donald Van De Veer (Belmont, Calif.: Wadsworth Publishing Company, 1988), pp. 49–55.

41. Mary O. Amdur, John Doull, and Curtis D. Klassen, eds., *Casaretti and Doull's Toxicology, The Basic Science of Poisons*, 4th ed. (London: Pergamon Press, 1991), pp. 31–33. Original literature citation is R. L. Hall, *Proceedings of Marabou Symposium on Foods and Cancer* (Stockholm: Castlan Press, 1979).

42. Kopelman, "Female Circumcision," p. 249–59.

43. U.S. Dietary Supplement Health and Education Act of 1994.

BONNIE B. O'CONNOR

Personal Experience, Popular Epistemology, and Complementary and Alternative Medicine Research

Now that the conventional medical and research establishments have begun to take complementary medicine seriously as a topic of investigation, it will behoove us to be mindful of—and active in—the ways in which the research agenda is developed and carried forward. As currently configured, this agenda reflects several well-articulated propositions: for example, that selected complementary and alternative medicine (CAM) systems and modalities should be evaluated for safety and efficacy, that "official" system representatives should oversee and be the primary executors of CAM research, that quantitative methods and carefully controlled clinical trials are the most desirable and reliable methods for conducting CAM research, that such research can accurately and reliably discover what works, and that modalities found by these means to be truly beneficial should be incorporated, where possible, into the conventional system's therapeutic armamentarium.[1] An unspoken accompanying assumption seems to be that those parts of the multimodal CAM domain that do not become scientifically validated as a result of this investigative effort over the next several years will not only fade from medical and scientific interest but will (or should) lose favor with the public as well, and that use of CAM healing resources that do not become officially sanctioned will (or should) then diminish accordingly.

While this model provides a framework for much that is of potential benefit to the research effort and its clinical applications, it is also limited in ways that are likely to compromise the value, and sometimes the validity, of many of the findings produced under its aegis. The model is scientistic, strongly medicocentric, and ultimately assimilationist. Its extreme one-sidedness sharply limits the kinds of research questions likely to be asked (and thus the kinds of knowledge that can be gleaned) and makes the model resistant to the methodological innovation that for such a novel and challenging subject seems both pressing and fitting. Perhaps its most serious omission is its failure to incorporate the self-identified needs, therapeutic goals, rationales, perspectives, experiences, and authoritative knowledge of the very public whose extensive and enthusiastic use of complementary medicine has propelled this topic into medical researchers' attention in the first place.

With a handful of notable exceptions, inclusion of the CAM-using public themselves in CAM research thus far has been largely to problematize their use of CAM and "diagnose" their motivations for using it. In its strong form, this is a classic positivist approach—a sort of "sociology of error"[2]—that takes medical and scientific norms at face value and aims to discover why, in the face of the advances and successes of modern biomedicine, people would want to seek care outside the conventional domain. This view assumes that conventional medical and scientific knowledge are (or should be) authoritative, that conventional medical care is (or should be) sufficient to the health care needs of patients, and that the health care pluralism represented by the public's recourse to CAM therapies therefore stands in need of explanation.

Often those explanations have been offered in social or psychological terms that have made attributions about patients (e.g., desperation, ignorance, irrationality, high control needs, and high rates of dissatisfaction with conventional medicine) that—when checked with CAM users themselves—have proved not to be the case for the substantial majority.[3] Approaching the question from the point of view of patients reveals that people typically seek complementary modalities for practical, problem-solving reasons: they have health needs that go beyond what conventional medicine does or can provide,[4] they wish to multiply their preventive and therapeutic options,[5] they have reason to believe these therapies may be useful, and/or they have philosophical and experiential reasons to find them attractive and reasonable choices.[6] Recent survey research finds that while CAM users tend to report generally poorer health status—a strong motivator for seeking additional prospects for health improvement—they cannot accurately be characterized as "desperate," and they do not demonstrate higher control needs or greater dissatisfaction with conventional medicine than the general public.[7]

Coming to Complementary Medicine: Two Cases

The following two case synopses, drawn from my ethnographic fieldwork with users of complementary medicine over the years, illustrate a few themes and patterns commonly found in this population. Each describes an educated, middle-class person in his or her initial foray into a practitioner-based complementary medicine system. Both of these individuals had on previous occasions used some self-prescribed vitamins, herbal supplements, or home remedies as a part of routine self-care, and one had experimented with a few homeopathic products. Each tended to purchase such items in "health foods" or natural foods stores because of market availability at the time. Neither considered such activity to be a departure from the ordinary or an intentional search for "another way" of approaching health issues. Rather, these products were part of the general and diverse over-the-counter inventory in these individuals' homes and of their conceptual frameworks for dealing with everyday health matters.

At the times represented in these narratives, both people were seeking to broaden their available range of therapeutic options for dealing with a troublesome health problem, and each was philosophically and practically disposed to experiment with "other ways" and observe the results. Each achieved a specific therapeutic goal, as well as more general therapeutic benefits, which he or she attributed to the CAM intervention. In each case, the individuals' combined and comparative experiences with both the conventional and complementary systems brought about fundamental and long-term changes in their health-related knowledge, belief, and practice. Neither rejected conventional medicine, though both, over time, came to see it as only one among several important and valid health care resources. Neither believes he or she will ever again find conventional medicine alone sufficient to address adequately issues of prevention, active health maintenance, or any significant challenges or compromises to health.

Case 1: Dr. David Nichols

David Nichols, age forty-two, is an executive in an urban business firm. His credentials include two advanced degrees, both earned at Ivy League universities. His professional position frequently requires him to conduct research and literature reviews, at which he is skilled, and he is in frequent demand as a speaker and trainer in his areas of expertise nationally. He has comprehensive health benefits, which allow him maximum personal choice and extensive coverage.

Dr. Nichols experiences a baffling febrile illness of sudden onset. It is characterized by cyclic dramatic rises in temperature to peaks of 101 to 103 degrees with accompanying profound fatigue and inability to concentrate, followed by breaks in the fevers accompanied by exhaustion, soaking perspiration, and deep sleep from which he awakens after an hour or so feeling alert and clear-headed but not refreshed. The cycles are approximately six hours in duration, and continue around the clock; the onset phase of the fevers frequently awakens him when it occurs during the night. During the second week of this pattern, Dr. Nichols begins to find himself unable to fully carry out the responsibilities of his job and has to cancel or hand off to colleagues several upcoming meetings and speaking engagements.

At this point Dr. Nichols seeks the advice of an infectious disease (ID) specialist of excellent reputation, who sees him immediately and begins a series of diagnostic tests. Dr. Nichols is put on prescription nonsteroidal antiinflammatory drugs (NSAIDs) in an attempt to control the fevers. By the end of the third week of the illness, testing has ruled out many possible diagnoses but confirmed none; symptoms continue as before. Dr. Nichols receives a diagnosis of FUO—"fever of unknown origin." His physician explains that treatment will be symptomatic pending a more specific diagnosis, but that there are many idiosyncratic viral diseases for which a definitive diagnosis may not emerge: "It may be that, in the end, the best we can say is that you had a typical case of 'Nichols's Disease.' "

The illness continues to interfere with Dr. Nichols's job and his home life, and its toll in fatigue and debilitation is cumulative. His medical treatment has only minor success. Other than reducing his peak temperatures to about 100 to 101 degrees, the NSAIDs do not provide relief from the cyclical fevers or their accompanying symptoms, and they make Dr. Nichols feel "like a pressure cooker with the lid on too tight." His subjective sensation is of two opposing forces (the fevers and the NSAIDs) pushing against each other in his body, which is their containment vessel. He feels that the drug is "putting a lid on" the fevers, but neither stopping them nor addressing their cause; the internal sensation of "pressure," an apparent effect of the NSAIDs, adds to his discomfort, in effect becoming an additional symptom.

Based on the reports of friends and acquaintances who have had personal successes with the system, Dr. Nichols decides he would like to try acupuncture and other aspects of traditional Chinese medicine (TCM) to treat his illness. He discusses this option with his physician, whose knowledge he respects and whose efforts he deeply appreciates. The physician is encouraging and offers to recommend a couple of medical acupuncturists, but Dr. Nichols demurs. He explains that he prefers to find someone trained in TCM and its underlying theoretical models since "how you go about defining a problem has a lot to do with what kinds of things suggest themselves as solutions." He also wishes to continue to see his ID specialist, who is agreeable to this plan.

By the end of the fourth week of his illness, Dr. Nichols begins treatment with a TCM practitioner, whose credentials include education at a U.S. school of oriental medicine, licensure in the state to practice acupuncture, and certification by the NCCA (National Center for the Certification of Acupuncturists, a professional peer review and certification body). His therapies include acupuncture and individualized prescriptions of Chinese herbs, furnished as dried herb mixtures, which he boils and prepares as a tea. He receives acupuncture once a week for ten to twelve weeks, and subsequently at longer intervals (two to three weeks). He experiences an appreciable reduction in symptom severity within the first week of TCM therapies and complete remission of the febrile cycles within three to four weeks. He continues to pursue TCM to rebuild his health and strength back to their pre-illness levels.[8]

Dr. Nichols's ID specialist had explained to him that most viral diseases of the type he believed his patient had contracted are self-limiting and will remit irrespective of treatment after an unpredictable period of time. In the absence of a known or treatable infectious agent, therapeutic interventions in the interim are designed to provide symptom relief. Nichols did not disbelieve this medical explanation. At the same time, he did not feel satisfied to restrict himself to a therapeutic course that could not address causes, did not attempt to strengthen his body's resources for handling the disease, and yielded poor results in symptom management. Nor did he feel willing to accept without further exploration a diagnostic framework that provided only a nonspecific, default diagnostic endpoint. In a recent interview, Dr. Nichols recalled that "the [big unanswered] question in Western terms was 'is it acute, or is it chronic?' I figured I had to hedge against the chronicity. I knew I had something that was patterned. Allopathic medicine couldn't give me a description, and the treatment wasn't adequate because of the 'pressure-cooker' thing."[9]

Dr. Nichols credited the acupuncture and Chinese herbs with the remission of his illness on the basis of observations of his subjective sensations in response to the therapeutic interventions of the TCM therapies and the conventional NSAIDs. The drug seemed regularly to produce unpleasant inner sensations of "suppression" or "pushing down" against the febrile cycles, while his immediate postacupuncture responses brought sensations of both physical and mental relief and release. Nichols had no prior expectations for TCM as he lacked knowledge of the system, apart from a general sense gleaned from friends that it was "good for" chronic problems. Thus it is unlikely that his experiences of acupuncture and its immediate sequelae were conditioned by a prior belief about what should happen. Rather, the experiences and sensations themselves (with both the conventional and the complementary therapies) began to shape a new understanding of illness and its treatment, particularly in terms of addressing symptoms by "opposing" them, rather than addressing underlying causes by making changes in causal conditions. These emergent views were consonant with TCM theories and thus received both theoretical reinforcement from that system as well as subjective ratification from Dr. Nichols's experiences and inner sensations.

Moving beyond the boundaries of conventional medicine did not diminish David Nichols's interest in or desire for access to skilled Western medical and scientific thinking. He felt he was getting this benefit in good measure from a physician who had his trust and respect and whom he wished to continue to see. Rather, Nichols sought to expand his total frame of reference by recruiting an entirely new diagnostic and therapeutic perspective. This, he felt, gave him the benefit of two complex and sophisticated conceptual schemata to bring to bear on his health care problem-solving efforts. In retrospect, he feels that TCM was able, through a combination of therapeutic interventions, to address his immediate needs in terms of symptom relief, the systemic imbalances that had created the conditions for the febrile disease to befall him, and the long-term health maintenance needs that would prevent further incidents of this type.

As of this writing, David Nichols continues to use TCM as his primary prevention and health maintenance system. He takes Chinese herbs daily and receives occasional acupuncture treatments on a "tune-up" basis. His success with TCM raised his interest in exploring other systems, and he has in recent years used occasional chiropractic treatments, therapeutic massage, and bodywork to beneficial effect. He also sees an internist annually for a physical exam and routine screenings. At fifty, he feels he has never been healthier in his life, seldom even coming down with a cold, and he feels he owes this to his continued active pursuit of Chinese medicine. For any serious health challenge, he would consult a physician as well as a TCM practitioner, and other modalities and providers if they seemed to be indicated. It is important to Dr. Nichols that his primary physician be open to his use of these complementary systems. Ideally, the physician would also be knowledge-able about them: "It would help me if he were able to take on more of a coordinating role, to help me manage across systems." If his physician is not able or comfortable to do so, however, "I wouldn't let it stop me; I'd just have to do it myself."[10]

Case 2: Dr. Katherine Davis

Dr. Katherine Davis, a faculty member at a large private East Coast university, goes to see an acupuncturist to discuss whether this modality might be beneficial in helping to deal with recurrent posterior tibial tendonitis and chronic foot and ankle pain of several years' duration. Though seldom severe, the pain is now nearly constant and has begun to interfere with sleep and with several of Dr. Davis's favorite recreational activities. Occasional steroid injections at inflammation sites have provided temporary relief only, and she has found NSAIDs ineffective for pain control, while producing unacceptable gastric side effects. In the past six years Dr. Davis has consulted three sports medicine orthopedists but has had disappointing results in spite of adopting a program of strengthening exercises and daily use of custom-fitted orthotics and supportive shoes.

During the past year, Dr. Davis has also experienced several episodes of minor, recurrent lower back discomfort that appears to be associated with onset of symptoms suggestive of incipient urinary tract infection, which typically flare briefly and then remit without intervention within the same day. In addition, she has had several months of very annoying, though not incapacitating, near-continuous upper respiratory symptoms suggestive of an adult-onset asthma or reactive airway disease. She has seen her primary physician (an internist) and one pulmonologist about these two sets of symptoms, which were not found to warrant therapeutic intervention. Dr. Davis does not consider these health events to be related, except through the possible mechanism of stress: she feels she has been generally "run down" because of work-related overcommitment and insuf-ficient "down time," leading to a general state of lowered resistance. None of this is on her mind as she speaks with the acupuncturist about her foot and ankle pain, which Dr. Davis considers "mechanical" in origin.

In the course of their discussion, the acupuncturist elicits this history as she asks Dr. Davis several questions about her general health, other troublesome symptoms, "constitutional weaknesses," or types of health disruption to which she seems particularly susceptible, and so forth. The acupuncturist says she does think that acupuncture will help with the chronic pain and tendonitis, and that it will address Dr. Davis's other symptoms as well. She explains that it is common to see these kinds of symptoms (foot/ankle, urinary, and upper respiratory) cluster together because "all of these problems lie on the Kidney Meridian," which a diagram in the office shows as passing through the lungs and the kidneys/lower back, as well as along the posterior tibial tendon. In the TCM nosology, she explains, this symptom cluster is indicative of a recognized syndrome arising from deficiencies in "kidney qi."

Dr. Davis is stunned to hear the practitioner identify a common diagnostic category in TCM which has no counterpart in conventional biomedicine, and which describes and provides an explanatory framework (though entirely novel to Dr. Davis) that encompasses not only her immediate problem but also other bothersome symptoms that she had heretofore considered to be concurrent but unrelated.[11]

Although Dr. Davis had read about traditional Chinese medicine prior to this time, she was not knowledgeable about it and was using a largely biomechanical conceptual framework in her discussion with the acupuncturist. In turning to acupuncture, she was seeking what she felt was a novel and potentially effective form of physical therapy to treat a specific, isolated orthopedic problem. She hoped that she might be able to obtain both symptomatic relief and possible longer-term preventive benefits. Having her other symptoms brought into the discussion surprised her. However, having them matter-of-factly recognized as being linked to her chief complaint as part of a well-recognized syndrome with a diagnostic name, explanation, and indicated therapeutic course was "a galvanizing moment" for Dr. Davis.[12]

Dr. Davis was familiar with holistic theories about health and illness and subscribed to them herself in a vague way. At the time, however, she conceived of her own health issues essentially in two parallel explanatory models:[13] a "mechanical" model for her long-term orthopedic problems, and an association of her other, more recent symptoms with mental and physical stress that she hypothesized resulted in possible lowered resistance to infectious agents or heightened susceptibility to irritants. The cognitive experience of her "galvanizing moment" quite suddenly gave Dr. Davis a new perspective on her own health problems; on conventional medicine and its analytical subdivision and separation of aspects of the body and its health; and on the radically divergent conceptual framework of traditional Chinese medicine, which she could now ground in her personal health experience.

Over the course of one month of weekly and two months of biweekly acupuncture treatments, which involved needling at various points on her body, Dr. Davis achieved good pain control in her feet and ankles, although she continued to experience occasional exacerbations following strenuous activity. She continued to pursue acupuncture for some eighteen months at biweekly to monthly intervals, during which time her tendonitis ceased to recur and her other symptoms also resolved. She did not pursue the Chinese herbs that her practitioner recommended as part of a complete therapeutic program because she found them too distasteful. To avoid their unpleasantness, she was willing to settle for what her practitioner warned her would be a longer time frame for achieving her preventive and therapeutic goals.

Dr. Davis discontinued her regular use of acupuncture at just short of two years, feeling that her therapeutic goals had been met and her gains consolidated. As of this writing she sees her primary care physician, an internist, annually for a physical exam and screenings and consults her at other times when she has a specific health problem that needs immediate attention. It is crucial to her that her physician is open to and knowledgeable about basic complementary modalities and willing and able to discuss them and to integrate them into her medical knowledge and thinking. Dr. Davis doubts she would remain in the care of a physician who did not evince these qualities. She uses vitamin and herbal supplements as part of her routine health maintenance regimen along with prescription medications as indicated. Since her initial favorable experience with acupuncture, she has continued to use it as a resource whenever she has had multiple concurrent health problems, which she considers, on the basis of her prior experiences, to be an indication of a state of internal imbalance which conventional medicine neither recognizes nor has the capacity to address.

Personal Experience and Popular Epistemology

Personal experience with health and illness, and with conventional and complementary medicine, interacts with individuals' philosophical and cognitive frameworks in a number of ways, as the cases cited demonstrate. For users of CAM, neither the criteria for defining health and illness nor those for defining valid knowledge about these matters are ceded entirely to licensed professionals.[14] Many accept "human experience [as] a valid way of knowing" and regard "the body as a source of reliable knowledge,"[15] rejecting the "assumption that personal experiences must be secondary to professional judgment."[16] This matter-of-fact lay empiricism stands in sharp contrast to scientific insistence that in the absence of technical expertise and controlled conditions our untrained observations are untrustworthy and potentially misleading.[17]

Knowledge that originates in the experiences and sensations of the body gives rise to a "practical epistemology," or pragmatic knowledge base, whose "standard of validity [is precisely] the question: Does it work? or Is it useful?"; that is, does it help "solve the problem [I am living with]?"[18] Scientific information is widely sought and valued but may not be accorded final authority. Rather, it is taken under advisement, much as one would do with advice from a professional consultant, and factored into decision making alongside other sources of information. Personal experiences of illness and healing carry significant evidentiary weight. If unacknowledged or contested by conventional medicine because of incongruities with medically accepted facts, personal experience may in fact trump medical/scientific claims and be considered the ultimate source of authoritative knowledge.[19]

People with chronic illnesses have long observed that they acquire "intimate understanding of [their] bodies and an acute sensitivity to changes in bodily function," which provide "an accurate and important source of information regarding the management of [their] condition[s]."[20] Similarly, it is common for users of complementary medicine to attend closely to their bodies and sensations, to say that they "listen to their bodies" in making health-related decisions, or to assert that "they know their own body best and trust their own judgment most."[21]

Conceptual Models

CAM users often hold conceptual models of health and illness and of physiological and psychological processes that depart in important ways from the conventional biomedical model, typically by expanding on it. These models may precede their exposure to CAM (and so perhaps predispose them to its use)[22] or may be a consequence of their experiences with complementary medicine bringing about cognitive and conceptual change. Most people who have cultural exposure to medical and scientific knowledge about the body—although clearly in laypersons' terms—do accept basic biological knowledge and theory. Significant numbers, however, find biology insufficient to explain their own complex health and illness experiences adequately and so do not restrict their understanding to a strictly biological conceptual schema.[23] Biological models are not necessarily rejected but are rather assessed as being underinclusive, as failing to account for crucial aspects of persons and their health that have wide public acceptance on both theoretical and experiential grounds.[24] These aspects include spiritual matters, self-healing capabilities of the body, and various forms of animating and regulatory vital energies.

Conceptions of the body are intimately interconnected with definitions of health and illness, with constructions of disease etiology, and with corollary notions of appropriate care. The nonbiomedical conceptualizations of the body and of health found in CAM systems resonate strongly, both philosophically and experientially, for large numbers of people. It is common, for example, for individuals to report that a given CAM modality or system and its approaches to healing are in important ways "more congruent with [their] experience of the body"[25] than what they have found in conventional medicine, or that they address personally critical aspects of their health and illness experiences that are not covered in the biomedical model. (Both of the people whose cases are presented above, for example, had such experiences.) These systems also typically accept individuals' personal experiences and observations as valid sources of clinically relevant knowledge. This concordance of CAM theory and practice with popular ontology and epistemology, or understandings of bodily reality and ways of knowing, helps to account for public acceptance and popularity of complementary medicine on grounds of both personal belief and direct personal experience.[26]

Are CAM Users "Antiscience"?

Neither these departures from conventional scientific and medical models nor the relativization of scientific and medical authority makes CAM enthusiasts "antiscience"—although that is an accusation frequently leveled at them in the conventional medical and research arenas. Perhaps some small percentage actually are, but my own research and that of others do not support this contention with respect to CAM users as a whole. Indeed, CAM users who are activists—either on their own behalf, in dealing with a specific health problem, or on behalf of the "cause" of CAM—tend to figure prominently among those who press for scientific investigation of CAM therapies. (In fact, they have done so since long before such suggestions were met with even the remotest acceptance in the medical and scientific communities.) In so doing, they assert their recognition of the cultural authority of science and seek to recruit it to the cause of complementary medicine—both as a means to its validation and legitimization and as a source of reliable information to facilitate public decision making about CAM use.

The following responses to a query about the value of scientific research on CAM that I recently posted on CAM-related Internet sites are representative of the general sentiment on the subject I have found repeatedly over eighteen years of ethnographic fieldwork on CAM and its users:

- From MB, female, moderator of an ADD/ADHD online forum: "I have been using alternative methods for over 4 years now. I highly believe in research and maintaining strict compliance with the FDA and the [DSHEA] act. . . . I also advocate using alternative methods instead of pharmaceuticals if at all possible for ADD."
- From RF, male, a university faculty member in psychology: "I am an occasional user of 'alternative' medicines and very much interested in science. . . . I pay a huge amount of attention to scientific literature. There are a lot of interesting substances out there that deserve scientific attention."
- From CG, female (no further information offered): "Clinical studies on supplements would be most beneficial . . . since the remedies might be proven."
- From BK, male, biochemist and cancer patient: "There is a tremendous need for studies to validate or refute the multitude of [CAM] therapies available, especially in the area of cancer treatment. I hear from so many who are confused by the vast number of options available to them. They are forced to make life or death decisions based on anecdote, here say [sic], and biased info from marketers and others with vested interests. Most of these people are crying out for valid studies to use in their selection process."
- From SW, male, parent of an adolescent with cystic fibrosis: "If it is asking the right questions. It's important. [sic]"

Similar views were repeatedly expressed by women interviewed by Wooddell and Hess about their use of complementary modalities as part of their cancer treatment regimens.[27] Medical and scientific knowledge is valued, but it is also recognized to have potential limitations in its applicability to the complexities of everyday life or its acceptability to one's own situation.[28] As one cancer patient reported about her assessment of medical treatment advice: "I always listen to my doctor, but I always weigh what he says and the second opinion is always my opinion."[29]

CAM users also express caution regarding the potential motives and putative fairness of scientific studies of CAM. Any potential that a study may be motivated by interests in profit or other personal or professional gain on the part of the researcher or the sponsor casts the results of the study into serious doubt—whether the results are favorable or unfavorable to CAM. (Nor is this judgment reserved exclusively for research on CAM: this sense of caution applies equally to studies on conventional pharmaceuticals.) Studies that seem designed to further a rhetorical agenda, either to discredit or to "push" a particular therapy, are met with similar skepticism. To all studies and results, the personal experience, personal trust, and personal judgment criteria are evaluatively applied. For example:

- From BK, Internet respondent: "Whether justified or not, there is a lot of skepticism that studies are designed to discredit various therapies. This is especially true in situations where large numbers of successful anecdotes [sic] contradict study findings. B-17 (laetrile) comes to mind as an example."
- From CG, Internet respondent: "[Scientific data matter.] Quite a bit. Especially when that data is filtered by a care giver I have chosen as our healthcare practitioner, which implies I trust his/ her judgment, not necessarily the information. . . . Healthcare giver advice usually has the most weight, then there are anecdotes of trusted friends and family, plus [my own] study on the compound and its generally understood action in the body. . . . Also, my own previous experience with the supplement."

CAM users clearly do "accept science as a key resource" in providing useful information about complementary modalities, but they do not necessarily "[accept] its authority in framing what the issues are"[30] or accord it undisputed epistemological status. Charging CAM users with being anti-scientific "when in fact they may simply [approach and apply] science in a nontraditional manner"[31] factually misrepresents the relationship these laypeople have with science. This imputation implies a critique of CAM users' rationality that has not been shown to be well founded, and it obscures the significant social fact that scientific pronouncements and agenda-setting "may legitimately be rejected [by members of the public] on grounds different from technical ignorance" or faulty judgment.[32]

Ironically, in fact, many members of the CAM-using public—as well as of activist groups of patients dealing with currently or recently "contested diseases" such as environmental illness/multiple chemical sensitivity[33] or repetitive strain injury,[34] or with contested therapeutic claims such as the greater effectiveness of smoked marijuana versus its pharmaceutical derivatives for controlling AIDS-related wasting syndromes—could well invert the "anti-science" accusation. Finding compelling and pragmatically useful knowledge in personal experiences of both illness and healing that the scientific community dismisses when approached for explanations or assistance, these are people who could defensibly claim that it is science that is rejecting them, and not the other way around.

Finding Out What Works

Medical researchers and laypeople who use CAM have different needs, goals, conceptual frameworks, and methods for producing and applying knowledge. Although very broadly, they share a genuine concern with finding out "what works," CAM users and scientific researchers generally have very different conceptualizations of what may be counted as "working," of what kinds of explanations are viable, and of what additional knowledge requirements are attached to the enterprise of testing and determining these things. For example, positing a plausible biological mechanism of action or maintaining theoretical consistency with existing scientific knowledge in their explanatory and conceptual models is generally of little or no concern to ordinary individuals seeking tangible health results in the context of their everyday lives.

Such differential goals and interests have long been recognized as a source of strain between the scientific community and its assertions about health claims on the one hand, and on the other hand the general public, which is far more likely to attach value to individual and collective health significance in real-life contexts than to statistical significance in controlled, artificial contexts. People concerned with the health effects of possible toxic exposures, for example, do not find utility in scientific assessments of the "probability of nonrandomness of an incident of illness" in their environs.[35] Rather, they seek a gauge of risk in personally meaningful, experientially grounded terms, such as "the likelihood that a reasonable person, including [a scientist] . . . would take up residence with the community . . . and drink from and bathe in the water from the Yellow Creek area or buy a house along Love Canal."[36] Cancer patients may define efficacy in terms of contributions to "long-term survival and quality of life, rather than tumor regression or short-term remission with poorer quality of life."[37] AIDS treatment activists stress their need to know how therapeutic agents will perform in the kinds of combinations and circumstances in which they will actually be taken by people with HIV disease (including multiple pharmaceuticals and complementary therapies used simultaneously), not merely how they will perform in tightly controlled trials of single agents.[38]

In complementary and alternative medicine also, the public want this type of practical, directly applicable knowledge from science. In addition, CAM users as a group assert a strong claim to the existence of medically novel types of benefits recognized through individual and collective experience. Many of the therapeutic effects of CAM modalities that laypeople seek and value are not recognized as valid in the conventional paradigm; others are defined as "nonspecific," rendering them unattributable to particular modalities or interventions, or nonamenable to study using typical quantitative research designs and extant scientific standards. Examples include subjectively noted improvements in general vigor or sense of well-being, promotion of active wellness,[39] support of the immune system[40] or of an inherent recuperative capacity of the body,[41] restoration of internal states of balance or harmony, spiritual benefits, or restoration of proper flow and function of qi or other vital energies. This disjunction poses a special challenge to CAM research, one that should not be overlooked.

Methodological and Epistemological Considerations

In the pursuit of the CAM research agenda to date, lay ontologies and epistemologies have consistently been effaced or discarded when they do not map "properly" onto scientific and medical categories. They need instead to be included in the definitions of research problems and responded to as valid and broadly shared viewpoints that provide crucial information about needs, goals, and experiences in patient populations. An overfocus on objective measures of narrowly defined efficacy will obscure many other important and clinically relevant aspects of complementary medicine. Not least of these are individuals' experienced needs in coping with illness and seeking to restore, maintain, and enhance health and intense public interest in therapeutic options whose features, and many of whose target outcomes, depart significantly from those of existing conventional treatments. Exploring the meanings that health, illness, and care have for ordinary people is essential to understanding a range of health behavior.[42] Many of these phenomena are accessible only to qualitative methodologies, which have the openness and flexibility to discover "indigenous" cognitive and experiential frameworks, and

CAM users' framing of the significant issues. Others will require development of new methodological approaches that can accommodate the multidimensionality of real-life practices and settings and investigate novel and "nonspecific" claims.

It is clear enough that "non-expert life experience can in fact locate and make sense of important facts about health."[43] This has been demonstrated many times and has on several occasions received scientific confirmation.[44] People who live with specific health problems have both self-identified needs and tangible, experiential knowledge that is "otherwise inaccessible to scientists" and that often "precedes official and scientific knowledge,"[45] and it can be an important spur to inquiry. This should be borne in mind in the identification of CAM research questions and methods—and in more innovative ways than simply identifying "most-used" substances and interventions in order to test them for efficacy. Laypeople's experiences of effects outside the range of scientific familiarity or statistical significance ought to pique our interest, even if difficult to investigate. (For example, the finding reported by Tom Whitmarsh in this volume of a trial of a homeopathic headache remedy in which the active intervention group [but not the placebo group] reported—in blinded interviews—that they had "felt better," even though objective measures found the tested remedy no more effective than placebo, is quite provocative. Is this a random artifact, or have these particular subjects possibly shared an experience of a type of effect that they and other patients value, but that researchers heretofore have missed?)

Sociologists of science have demonstrated convincingly and frequently that "deficit theories" of incongruities of lay knowledge claims and behaviors with the knowledge claims and prescriptions of science are often incorrect and usually counterproductive, both for the public and for the community of scientists.[46] Medicocentrism, the defining of issues from the medical viewpoint to the exclusion of the viewpoints of patients, has led to mischaracterization of such important phenomena as adherence behavior[47] and the very persistence, appeal, and steadily increasing popularity of CAM itself over the last few decades. It is important not to perpetuate this error in pursuing CAM research now, or the best we can hope for is an "official" picture of complementary medicine that ultimately has an imperfect and deceptive bearing on how and why these therapies are actually used so widely.

The task of investigating complementary and alternative medicine and understanding its patterns of use and utility is complex and is a focal point for tensions between lay and professional knowledge-making claims and assertions of authority. It also holds potential to provide a meeting ground on which differential claims may become mutually illuminating (rather than merely competing) and a field in which methodological innovation may make significant strides. If the scientific research agenda for CAM is to be of significant interest and value to the public, then the research must address the concerns of that public as well as the concerns of scientists and clinicians. And if we are going to seek some integration in conventional settings—a move for which there is clearly public and institutional support[48]—it cannot be accomplished simply by appropriating and medicalizing selected therapeutic modalities. Rather, a truly *integrative* approach to health care will have to accommodate multiple conceptual and healing models, effectively combine qualitative and quantitative research methodologies, and give weight to patient as well as professional interests, problem definitions, and outcome measures.

NOTES

1. David J. Hufford, "Culturally Grounded Review of Research Assumptions," *Alternative Therapies in Health and Medicine* 2, no. 4 (1996): 47–53.

2. Brian Martin and Eveleen Richards, "Scientific Knowledge, Controversy, and Public Decision Making," in *Handbook of Science and Technology Studies*, ed. Sheila Jasanoff et al. (Thousand Oaks, Calif.: Sage Publications, 1995), pp. 506–26, at 509.

3. David J. Hufford, "Contemporary Folk Medicine," in *Other Healers: Unorthodox Medicine in America,* ed. Norman Gevitz (Baltimore: Johns Hopkins University Press, 1988), pp. 228–64; Bonnie B. O'Connor, *Healing Traditions: Alternative Medicine and the Health Professions* (Philadelphia: University of Pennsylvania Press, 1995); John Astin, "Why Patients Use Alternative Medicine: Results of a National Study," *JAMA* 278, no. 19 (1998): 1548–53.

4. Hufford, "Contemporary Folk Medicine."

5. O'Connor, *Healing Traditions.*

6. Hufford, "Contemporary Folk Medicine"; Astin, "Why Patients Use Alternative Medicine"; Bonnie B. O'Connor, "Conceptions of the Body in Complementary and Alternative Medicine," in *Complementary Medicine: Challenge and Change,* ed. Merrijoy Kelner and Beverly Wellman (Reading, England: Harwood Academic Publishers, 2000), pp. 39–60.

7. Astin, "Why Patients Use Alternative Medicine."

8. David Nichols (pseudonym), ethnographic interviews and participant observation by author (multiple occasions), 1992.

9. Nichols, interview by author, May 2000.

10. Nichols, interview by author, May 2000.

11. Katherine Davis (pseudonym), ethnographic interviews and participant observation by author (multiple occasions), 1993.

12. Davis, personal journal, 1993.

13. Arthur Kleinman, "Explanatory Models in Health-Care Relationships," in *Health of the Family* (Washington, D.C.: National Council for International Health, 1975), pp. 159–72.

14. Lowell S. Levin, Alfred H. Katz, and Erik Holst, *Self-Care: Lay Initiatives in Health* (New York: Prodist, 1979); Bonnie B. O'Connor, "The Home Birth Movement in the United States," *Journal of Medicine and Philosophy* 18, no. 2 (1993): 147–74; Sarah Cant and Ursula Sharma, eds., *Complementary and Alternative Medicines: Knowledge in Practice* (London: Free Association Books, 1996); Mark A. Chesler, "Mobilizing Consumer Activism in Health Care: The Role of Self-Help Groups," *Research in Social Movements, Conflict and Change* 13 (1991): 275–305.

15. Steve Kroll-Smith and H. Hugh Floyd, *Bodies in Protest: Environmental Illness and the Struggle over Medical Knowledge* (New York: New York University Press, 1997), p. 118.

16. Kroll-Smith and Floyd, *Bodies in Protest*, p. 112.

17. Claire Cassidy, "Social Science Theory and Methods in the Study of Alternative and Complementary Medicine," *Journal of Alternative and Complementary Medicine* 1, no. 1 (1995): 19–40; Carol M. Davis, "Introduction," in *Complementary Therapies in Rehabilitation: Holistic Approaches for Prevention and Wellness,* ed. Carol M. Davis (Thorofare, N.J.: Slack, 1997), pp. xxix–xlv.

18. Kroll-Smith and Floyd, *Bodies in Protest,* p. 137.

19. Bonnie B. O'Connor, "The Authority of Experience and Beliefs about Knowing," paper presented to the American Folklore Society annual meeting, Cincinnati, Ohio, 1985; Kroll-Smith and Floyd, *Bodies in Protest*; O'Connor, "Conceptions of the Body in Complementary and Alternative Medicine."

20. S. Kay Toombs, "Chronic Illness and the Goals of Medicine," *Second Opinion* 21, no. 1 (1995): 11–19, at 13.

21. Merrijoy Kelner and Beverly Wellman, "Health Care and Consumer Choice: Medical and Alternative Therapies" *Social Science and Medicine* 45, no. 2 (1997): 203–12, at 210.

22. Astin, "Why Patients Use Alternative Medicine."

23. Espen Braathen, "Communicating the Individual Body and the Body Politic: The Discourse on Disease Prevention and Health Promotion in Alternative Therapies," in *Complementary and Alternative Medicines: Knowledge in Practice,* ed. Sarah Cant and Ursula Sharma (London: Free Association Books, 1996), pp. 151–62.

24. O'Connor, "Conceptions of the Body in Complementary and Alternative Medicine."

25. Helen Busby, "Alternative Medicines/Alternative Knowledges: Putting Flesh on the Bones (Using Traditional Chinese Approaches to Healing)," in *Complementary and Alternative Medicine,* pp. 135–50.

26. O'Connor, "Conceptions of the Body in Complementary and Alternative Medicine."

27. Margaret J. Wooddell and David J. Hess, *Women Confront Cancer: Making Medical History by Choosing Alternative and Complementary Therapies* (New York: New York University Press, 1998).

28. Alan Irwin and Brian Wynne, eds., *Misunderstanding Science? The Public Reconstruction of Science and Technology* (Cambridge, England: Cambridge University Press, 1996); Klaus Linde and Wayne B. Jonas, "Evaluating Complementary and Alternative Medicine: The Balance of Rigor and Relevance," in *Essentials of Complementary and Alternative Medicine,* ed. Wayne B. Jonas and Jeffrey S. Levin (Philadelphia: Lippincott Williams & Wilkins, 1999), pp. 57–71; Helen Lambert and Hilary Rose, "Disembodied Knowledge? Making Sense of Medical Science," in *Misunderstanding Science?* pp. 65–83; Chesler, "Mobilizing Consumer Activism in Health Care"; Linda M. Hunt et al., "Compliance and the Patient's Perspective: Controlling Symptoms in Everyday Life," *Culture, Medicine and Psychiatry* 13, no. 3 (1989): 315–34.

29. Wooddell and Hess, *Women Confront Cancer,* p. 191.

30. Alan Irwin and Brian Wynne, "Introduction," in *Misunderstanding Science?* pp. 1–18, at 8–9.

31. Phil Brown, "Popular Epidemiology and Toxic Waste Contamination: Lay and Professional Ways of Knowing," *Journal of Health and Social Behavior* 33 (September 1992): 267–81, at 276.

32. Brian Wynne, "Misunderstood Misunderstandings: Social Identities and Public Uptake of Science," in *Misunderstanding Science?* pp. 361–88, at 377.

33. Kroll-Smith and Floyd, *Bodies in Protest.*

34. Hilary Arksey, "Expert and Lay Participation in the Construction of Medical Knowledge," *Sociology of Health and Illness* 16, no. 4 (1994): 448–68.

35. Brown, "Popular Epidemiology and Toxic Waste Contamination," p. 274.

36. Brown, "Popular Epidemiology and Toxic Waste Contamination," p. 274.

37. David J. Hess, *Evaluating Alternative Cancer Therapies: A Guide to the Science and Politics of an Emerging Medical Field* (New Brunswick, N.J.: Rutgers University Press, 1999), p. 197.

38. Steven Epstein, *Impure Science: AIDS, Activism, and the Politics of Knowledge* (Berkeley: University of California Press, 1996).

39. Astin, "Why Patients Use Alternative Medicine."

40. Wooddell and Hess, *Women Confront Cancer.*

41. Busby, "Alternative Medicines/Alternative Knowledges."

42. Hunt et al., "Compliance and the Patient's Perspective."

43. David J. Hufford, comment at Hastings Center CAM working group meeting, Garrison, N.Y., December 12, 1999.

44. Arksey, "Expert and Lay Participation in the Construction of Medical Knowledge"; R. W. Spjut and R. E. Perdue, Jr., "Plant Folklore: A Tool for Predicting Sources of Antitumor Activity?" *Cancer Treatment Report* 60, no. 8 (1976): 979–85; E. Hilton et al., "Ingestion of Yogurt Containing Lactobacillus Acidophilus as Prophylaxis for Candidal Vaginitis," *Annals of Internal Medicine* 116, no. 5 (1992): 353–57; J. Avorn et al., "Reduction of Bacteriuria and Pyuria after Ingestion of Cranberry Juice," *JAMA* 271, no. 10 (1994): 751–54; G. L. Freed et al., "National Assessment of Physicians' Breast-Feeding Knowledge, Attitudes, Training, and Experience," *JAMA* 273, no. 6 (1995): 472–76.

45. Brown, "Popular Epidemiology and Toxic Waste Contamination," p. 270.

46. Irwin and Wynne, *Misunderstanding Science?*

47. Hunt et al., "Compliance and the Patient's Perspective"; James A. Trostle, W. Allen Hauser, and Ida S. Susser, "The Logic of Noncompliance: Management of Epilepsy from the Patient's Point of View," *Culture, Medicine and Psychiatry* 7 (1983): 35–56; Peter Conrad, "The Meaning of Medications: Another Look at Compliance," *Social Science and Medicine* 20, no. 1 (1985): 29–37; James A. Trostle, "Medical Compliance as an Ideology," *Social Science and Medicine* 27, no. 12 (1988): 1299–1308; Esther Sumartojo, "When Tuberculosis Treatment Fails: A Social Behavioral Account of Patient Adherence," *American Review of Respiratory Diseases* 147 (1993): 1311–20.

48. *The Landmark Report on Public Perceptions of Alternative Care* (Sacramento: Landmark Healthcare, 1998).

HOWARD BRODY

The Placebo Effect: Implications for the Study and Practice of Complementary and Alternative Medicine

The subject of complementary and alternative medicine (CAM) is insepa-
rable from that of the placebo effect (PE). It is difficult to engage in
conversation about CAM for more than five minutes among conventional
medical practitioners or investigators before one hears the question,
"How much of the effectiveness of CAM is due to the PE?" Opponents
of CAM raise this question largely to dismiss CAM. Supporters may
raise the question as a matter of genuine scientific curiosity, or as an
acknowledgment of the high level of enthusiasm displayed by many
CAM practitioners and recipients.

This chapter will first review some basic aspects of the PE and then
discuss some implications of the PE for both research and practice of
CAM. If there is a general theme that runs through the discussion, it
is that the gulf between CAM and conventional medicine—insofar as
this particular set of issues goes—may be much narrower than most
conventional medicine defenders like to think.

A paper that would be highly illuminating, but that has yet to be
written, is a history of U.S. academic medicine over the past thirty or
forty years, looking at the power struggle among three camps: conventional or "Flexnerian" academic medicine, primary care (including the
recent emergence of "evidence-based" medicine), and CAM. (Gail Geller
has suggested that one could add a fourth camp, bioethics, to this mix,
and that important parallels would be found.)[1] Many of the conceptual
and scientific issues I will address below are difficult to resolve precisely
because what may appear on the surface to be an intellectual conversation
is, underneath, a jockeying for a position of power—those currently
with power seeking to maintain their monopoly, and those without

power seeking to grab some. I do not believe it accidental that the evidence-based medicine movement and CAM have arisen on the traditional "turf" of conventional medicine, and have challenged its hegemony, at roughly the same point in history.

Preliminary Conceptual Issues

I will define *placebo effect* for our purposes as the bodily change due to symbolic effect of a treatment or treatment situation and not its pharmacologic or physiologic properties. By this definition, a PE may accompany an effect due to other causes as well, so that "drug" effects and PEs can exist side by side. Also by this definition, the PE can be either positive or negative in direction (so as to include so-called nocebo effects). This is a broad but not overly broad definition of PE. It excludes a good deal of what is often referred to as "mind-body healing." For example, if one engages in daily meditation, this may have positive health effects, but these would not be termed a PE. On the other hand, if believing strongly in the power of meditation enhanced the resulting effects, then that "added" enhancement could be legitimately called a PE.

One literature review that concluded that the PE, for the most part, does not exist depends heavily on a much narrower definition of PE: that it is the effect that results from administering sugar pills or other dummy treatments.[2] Those authors wished to admit that psychosomatic effects occur and indeed are extremely powerful, but they wished to distinguish those powerful mind-body interactions from PEs. I would defend the broader definition given above on two counts. First, as we will see momentarily, it is probable that the PE works via many of the same biochemical pathways as other mind-body interactions, so to insist that it is completely different in kind seems arbitrary. Second, those authors seem heavily influenced by concern over the negative connotations traditionally attached to the term PE (below). But there is no logically necessary connection between these connotations and the PE as I have defined it.

Two terms commonly used in definitions offered in the medical and psychological literature are *inert* and *nonspecific*. Neither is helpful and both are in fact misleading. Since the placebo stimulus, whatever it may be, by definition produces a bodily change, it can hardly be said to be inert. Also, since the PE is almost always in the direction predicted, based on the nature of the placebo stimulus, it can hardly be described as nonspecific. (That is, if a group of asthmatics are given a placebo and told it is a powerful medicine for asthma, a certain percentage of them will have improved respiratory function, peak flow, and so forth, but will *not* exhibit relief of pain, nausea, rashes, or other symptoms. By contrast, a group of sufferers from allergic rashes, given the same placebo and told it is a dermatologic remedy, may experience relief of itching and redness but not any improvement in breathing.)

It is easier to explain what the PE is not than to specify exactly what it is; and indeed, arguments have been offered as to the logical impossibility of defining PE in a completely consistent fashion.[3] The word "placebo" has, since medieval times, attracted negative connotations. Among the various negative associations are the following:

- *Deception:* the PE depends on a lie about what is being given; if people knew they were getting sugar pills they would derive no benefit.
- *Quackery:* only incompetent practitioners need to rely on a placebo; a properly trained practitioner would give the "real" medicine and effect a cure by that means.
- *Nuisance:* if a successful therapy is one that is superior to placebo in a double-blind, randomized controlled trial (RCT), then every occurrence of a PE makes it less likely that a promising therapy will be shown to be useful.
- *Mental:* medicine has traditionally privileged the body and devalued the mind, so any treatment that depends on mental processes is automatically suspect and viewed as less real.

Why do these negative connotations matter today? Many supposedly scientific views of the PE are biased by these connotations and so must be interpreted with caution—as in the case of the supposedly negative systematic review already mentioned.[4]

Preliminary Empirical Issues

For the purposes of this chapter I will assume two important things about the PE. First, I will assume that such a thing exists and is in fact a widespread phenomenon within human healing (whether by conventional medicine or CAM). The best evidence that this is so may be meta-analyses of more-than-two-armed RCTs and of the original, uncontrolled trials of therapies now universally regarded as useless.[5]

Second, I will assume that this effect probably operates at least in part via known psychosomatic biochemical pathways, including the endorphin, psychoneuroimmune, and catecholamine/cortisol pathways. Currently, no sets of data exist that trace a complete train of causation of the general form: symbolic stimulus in environment > interpretation by mind > biochemical pathway > end organ change. But there are highly suggestive, partial bits of evidence for portions of this causal chain, and it seems plausible that further research will reveal additional links.

The PE and the Study of CAM

One of the claims that must be critically assessed is: "The problem with our scientific understanding of CAM today is that most CAM modalities have not been carefully tested by RCTs. If they were, we'd understand whether any specific CAM modality really works or whether it is simply a form of placebo." This in turn requires a careful critical evaluation of the role of RCTs in medical science generally. RCTs have important limits that are often not well appreciated by either practicing physicians or medical scientists.

First, as a methodologist of my acquaintance once pointed out, an RCT is a very good way to find out, with a very high level of certainty, that very small differences are not due to chance. It is easy to forget that when major medical breakthroughs occurred, such as the introduction of insulin and penicillin, no one needed an RCT to demonstrate benefit.

Second, the RCT supposedly controls for all "nondrug" factors, but does so by lumping them all into the same wastebasket category so none of them are actually dissected out and studied. The RCT therefore assumes that every causative factor *except* for the "pure" drug or pharmacologic factor is of no interest whatever to the medical scientist. (We will see presently that the idea of the "pure" drug factor is probably a myth in any case.)[6]

Third, as a result of the latter point, the RCT assumes that the beliefs, thoughts, and meanings of the patient are worthy of neither attention nor study and exert no causal influence on the outcome of therapy that would be of interest to the scientist.

One way to approach the problem of studying CAM by means of RCTs is to investigate Barfod's notion of "fragility."[7] Basically, Barfod argues that various CAM modalities lie along a spectrum. At one end of the spectrum are treatments that most resemble the "ideal" conventional drugs in acting in a way quite independent of the patient's belief system or cultural environment. (Herbal remedies sold off the shelf in drugstores may exemplify this end of the spectrum.) At the other end are treatments whose effectiveness depends almost completely on the cultural context or belief system of practitioner and patient. (Faith-based systems such as Christian Science healing may be an example.) Thus the spectrum might be characterized as context/belief-independence at one end and context/belief-dependence at the other. Barfod refers to therapies at the latter end of the spectrum as "fragile" therapies. At the nonfragile end of the spectrum, the RCT is a legitimate and effective way to test the therapy scientifically, but as the therapy moves toward the fragile end, it becomes harder to view the RCT as a useful or fair method of assessment. Therapies that might be highly effective within the proper cultural and belief context might prove to be totally ineffective within the foreign environment required for and created by the conduct of an RCT. A research methodology more akin to naturalistic study or ethnographic field work would be required to study truly fragile treatments.

At first glance, the fragile-nonfragile spectrum seems to be descriptive of CAM but irrelevant to the study of conventional medicine. The fallacy of this view brings us back to the myth of the "pure" pharmacologic drug effect. Consider the following extended example.

Imagine that the drug for the treatment of erectile dysfunction, Viagra, has been tested under a variety of conditions. Imagine that we have an agreed-upon, reasonably objective measure of the successful treatment of erectile dysfunction. Imagine that the following data have been gathered in repeated, well-designed, and reproducible trials.

Condition of drug administration	Subjects improved, %
Viagra administered under "open label" conditions	90
Subject enrolled in double-blind RCT, told he will receive either Viagra or placebo; actually receives Viagra	70
Subject enrolled in double-blind RCT, told he will receive either an unnamed, "active" drug or placebo; actually receives Viagra	40
Viagra placed surreptitiously in subject's beverage or food	20

No such set of studies has been done to my knowledge, but the percentages indicated, as rough estimates, are plausible given existing data on the PE in various circumstances.[8]

Now the question arises: what is the "true" efficacy of Viagra? If the RCT is the scientific gold standard, then it would seem as if one of the two RCT results is the "right" answer. But which? The "open label" use resembles the conditions under which Viagra would be used therapeutically much more than either RCT does, so why is that not the better answer? Finally, if one's concern is with the "pure" pharmaco-logic drug effect, then it would seem that the surreptitious administration data is most pertinent; yet that usage is again extremely distant from any real clinical setting. The conclusion I would draw is that a conventional drug like Viagra is every bit as fragile as any CAM treatment.

This conclusion suggests that the RCT may do as poor a job of assessing at least some conventional remedies as it may in assessing at least some CAM remedies. Another way to put the point is that patient beliefs may exert a causal influence *within conventional medicine* that cannot and should not be eliminated from systematic scientific study.

This in turn raises a point about an important distinction that seems sometimes to be neglected by some advocates of evidence-based medicine—especially that variety of evidence-based medicine that amounts to a celebration of RCTs to the exclusion of any other sort of medical data. The distinction is between hypothetical and real RCTs. In theory, one could design an RCT to control for any variable and to study any variable (or, at least, the relative difference between any two variables). If I am trying to determine whether Drug A or Drug B is the better drug to give to my patient, I can, in theory, design an RCT involving one thousand subjects, all of whom are *just like my patient in all relevant ways,* five hundred of whom get Drug A and five hundred of whom get Drug B. By comparing the relevant clinical outcomes between the two groups I would have a high level of confidence as to which drug would be superior for my patient's use. In this hypothetical situation, patient beliefs offer no barrier to understanding; I could insist that we select one thousand subjects who share precisely the same beliefs about diseases and drugs as my patient has.

The problem, of course, is that while one could *hypothetically* design and conduct an RCT of this sort, it is extremely unlikely that any *real* RCT reported in the medical literature would have these features. At least some advocates for evidence-based medicine seem to be praising the RCT methodology based on what it is hypothetically capable of and then playing a sort of bait-and-switch by providing us with the results of real RCTs as if they held the answer to all clinical questions.

A stronger way of restating the relevant point is that each patient is a unique individual, and we possess no scientific method for applying data extracted from a population of somewhat similar individuals with absolute certainty to the individual case. Thus, conducting RCTs makes medicine "scientific" only in a limited sense. And that brings us to the question of the application of these considerations to clinical practice.

The PE and the Practice of CAM

If RCTs do not provide all the answers they first seemed to promise, then we could ask instead: what sorts of research into CAM will best identify those elements of the healing encounter and the administration of therapy that are most "placebogenic"? How can these elements then be further enhanced within the practice of CAM? And will it be possible to export at least some of those elements into conventional medicine, assuming, as thoughtful critics have noted, that it is precisely the absence of those features within much of conventional medicine today that has sparked the apparently immense public interest in CAM?[9]

It may seem at first that these elements of CAM would not be exportable, to the extent that what is principally responsible for whatever PE accompanies CAM is the mere fact that CAM *is not* conventional medicine—that it is "better" in some way, perceived as more exotic or more natural or whatever. But I submit that this answer is probably too simplistic. The reasons why people in the United States seek CAM are more complicated then the mere fact that CAM is not conventional medicine.[10] Careful study would be needed to answer the range of questions I have posed, which is beyond the scope of this chapter.

We then arrive at some of the most critical ethical questions relating to the role of PE in CAM. Again let me propose a thought experiment. Suppose that all of the following are true:

1. A certain CAM modality has been reported, in numerous observational studies, to be effective for treating the discomfort, and improving the function and quality of life, among sufferers from a form of chronic arthritis.

2. This modality is extensively studied and it is shown, as conclusively as possible, that its clinical effectiveness is due *totally* to the PE. Exhaustive study has revealed no other plausible explanation for its observed effects, and biochemical markers known to be associated with the PE are found to be consistently elevated following the use of this modality (e.g., endorphin levels).

3. No current conventional therapy treats this particular form and severity of arthritis as well as this CAM modality.

4. The group of sufferers from this form of arthritis (or, perhaps, a subset of them) are, for whatever reason, quite resistant to other stimuli that would ordinarily produce a PE. It seems that *only* this CAM modality is capable of eliciting a PE in this group (or subgroup).

The question then arises: assuming that the above facts are all carefully documented in the scientific medical literature, *should conventional physicians recommend this CAM treatment for that particular group of arthritis sufferers?* If the answer is "no," on what basis could that answer be given?

I can readily imagine the rejoinder, "Of course one would, under these circumstances, recommend that treatment. But at the same time one would insist that all such patients be fully and frankly informed that the CAM treatment is *nothing but* a placebo. To do otherwise would be to practice fraud upon our patients." One reply to the rejoinder is: "Suppose then that new, carefully designed empirical studies are carried out, and it turns out that when this group of sufferers goes through the 'informed consent' process just described, the efficacy of the treatment is reduced by 50 percent. Would one then still insist on frank disclosure? And if so, on what grounds?"

Another reply, perhaps more pertinent to our discussion, would be: "Are you also going to insist that every patient receiving a conventional remedy be fully and frankly informed as to the percentage of efficacy of that remedy that is due to the PE rather than to the 'pure' pharmacologic potency of the drug? If not, why not?" As the Viagra example shows, our best evidence today goes to show that the PE is a substantial portion or component of the efficacy of many conventional drugs and therapies.

Conclusion

Dr. Ted Kaptchuk, in discussions that were part of the project from which this book of essays emerged, may have projected the ultimate solution to the problem: replace the ethic of informed consent with the ethic of beneficence once again in medical practice. Let the medical scientists study causal mechanisms to their heart's content. Let all practitioners (CAM and conventional) administer treatments that seem to them and to the patients to work. All we need to do is to retrain the scientists away from the hubris of claiming that their data should govern the realm of medical practice in some privileged way.

Things, of course, are not quite so simple as that. There are important benefits to the ethic of informed consent and the respect for the rights and choices of patients on which it is based. Physicians trying merely to do "what seems to work" with beneficent intent have always wreaked, and continue to wreak, serious harm upon patients. One can in fact learn useful information from RCTs, and, on balance, it is probably somewhat better to base one's practice more on RCT results and less on what one was taught by one's senior mentor back in residency. Even though evidence-based medicine can be misused and misrepresented, there is a good deal of value in what it teaches us. And finally, when our present phase of excitement over CAM passes, it will no doubt have been shown to almost everyone's satisfaction that some of CAM, at least, is probably worthless, and even that some of it is harmful.

And so the more modest lesson that I would draw from the discussion of CAM and the PE is that the PE turns out to be quite a neutral concept in whatever battle might be fought between CAM and conventional medicine. Most criticisms of CAM, grounded in the PE, turn out on further study to be quite similar to criticisms that could equally well be lodged against conventional medicine.

I mentioned at the outset that I did not think it accidental that the evidence-based medicine and the pro-CAM "movements" seem to have arisen within conventional medicine at about the same time. Each movement, in its own way (but with some overlap), asks about the state of the wardrobe of the conventional-medicine emperor. To the extent that the emperor lays claim to being "scientific," he has no choice but to smile with approval at the various allegations of his nakedness. Even if these claims are not self-evidently true, investigating them is very likely to teach us a number of interesting things about the scientific basis of both conventional medicine and CAM.

NOTES

1. Gail Geller, "Assessment of Current Models" (paper presented at the conference Complementary and Alternative Therapies in the Academic Medical Center: Issues in Ethics and Policy, Philadelphia, Pa., November 10–12, 1999).

2. Gunver S. Kienle and Helmut Kiene, "Placebo Effect and Placebo Concept: A Critical Methodological and Conceptual Analysis of Reports on the Magnitude of the Placebo Effect," *Alternative Therapies* 2, no. 6 (1996): 39–54.

3. Peter C. Gøtzsche, "Is There Logic in the Placebo?" *The Lancet* 344 (October 1, 1994): 925–26; Irving Kirsch, "Unsuccessful Redefinitions of the Term *Placebo,*" *American Psychologist* 41 (July 1986): 844–45.

4. Kienle and Kiene, "Placebo Effect and Placebo Concept."

5. Jos Kleijnen et al., "Placebo Effect in Double-Blind Clinical Trials: A Review of Interactions with Medications," *The Lancet* 344 (November 12, 1994): 1347–49; Alan H. Roberts et al., "The Power of Nonspecific Effects in Healing: Implications for Psychosocial and Biological Treatments," *Clinical Psychology Review* 13 (1993): 375–91.

6. Seymour Fisher and Roger P. Greenberg, "The Curse of the Placebo: Fanciful Pursuit of a Pure Biological Therapy," in *From Placebo to Panacea: Putting Psychiatric Drugs to the Test,* ed. Seymour Fisher and Roger P. Greenberg (New York: John Wiley & Sons, 1997), pp. 3–56.

7. Toke Barfod, "Four Aspects of Placebo," in *Studies in Alternative Therapy 3: Communication in and about Alternative Therapies,* ed. Erling Høg and Søren Gosvig Olesen (Odense, Denmark: Odense University Press, 1996), pp. 111–26.

8. When new, highly touted treatments are used in "open label" situations, they may show extremely high efficacy, even in cases where double-blind studies later reveal the therapy to be useless: Roberts et al., "The Power of Nonspecific Effects in Healing." Subjects respond better to the "active" drug in a double-blind trial when they know that the other drug they might receive is another "active" drug rather than a placebo: Paula A. Rochon et al., "Are Randomized Controlled Trial Outcomes Influenced by the Inclusion of a Placebo Group? A Systematic Review of Nonsteroidal Antiinflammatory Drug Trials for Arthritis Treatment," *Journal of Clinical Epidemiology* 52 (February 1999): 113–22. Subjects respond better to tablets (whether placebo or aspirin) when marked with a well-known trade name than when the tablets are blank: A. Branthwaite and P. Cooper, "Analgesic Effects of Branding in Treatment of Headaches," *British Medical Journal* 282 (May 16, 1981): 1576–78. Subjects given either amphetamine or chloral hydrate, but no verbal cues as to what they were receiving, were unable to distinguish between the effects of those two drugs: S. B. Lyerly et al., "Drugs and Placebos: The Effects of Instruction upon Performance and Mood Under Amphetamine Sulphate and Chloral Hydrate," *Journal of Abnormal and Social Psychology* 68 (1964): 321–27.

9. Frank Davidoff, "Weighing the Alternatives: Lessons from the Paradoxes of Alternative Medicine," *Annals of Internal Medicine* 129 (December 15, 1998): 1068–70.

10. John A. Astin, "Why Patients Use Alternative Medicine: Results of a National Study," *JAMA* 279 (May 20, 1998): 1548–53; Ted J. Kaptchuk and David M. Eisenberg, "The Persuasive Appeal of Alternative Medicine," *Annals of Internal Medicine* 129 (December 15, 1998): 1061–65.

DAVID B. LARSON AND SUSAN S. LARSON

Spirituality in Clinical Care: A Brief Review of Patient Desire, Physician Response, and Research Opportunities

Patients' frequent use of "unconventional" or alternative medical treatments became well recognized through Eisenberg and his colleagues' national sample survey published in *The New England Journal of Medicine* in 1993. Yet, several of these survey findings remain less highlighted: some 25 percent of these patients used prayer during the previous year, 9 percent had sought out a spiritual healer, and 4 percent had utilized spiritual healing.[1]

How do these findings compare with the frequency of prayer or spiritual healing in other surveys of those suffering with illness or disabilities? Do many patients desire to incorporate recognition of their religious/spiritual values into their medical care? How aware are health care providers of the potential relevance of spiritual/religious factors in enhancing patient's coping or recovery? While a majority of U.S. medical schools now offer courses training future physicians in how to address a patient's spiritual framework, how often and how well are researchers in various medical fields investigating the impact of religious commitment on physical and mental health? This chapter will address these questions.

The Use of Prayer

Regarding the U.S. population, a substantial 90 percent of citizens pray at least occasionally, according to a Gallup poll. Most (97 percent) believe their prayers are heard, and 86 percent believe praying makes them better people.[2] Among patients, researchers in a recent review found that many use prayer to cope with life's problems, and that prayer may become an even greater personal resource as one's illness or disabilities become more serious.[3] This review extensively summarized who prays, why they pray, and the types of prayer used, and it reviewed the relevant clinical research findings to date.

Other studies have found that when patients are in psychiatric, medical, or surgical inpatient settings, between 80 and 90 percent would like to receive prayer, and more than 95 percent pray prior to cardiac surgery. Most of these patients perceive prayer to be an important factor in their achieving surgical success.[4] In a recent survey of arthritis patients, more than one-half (53 percent) used prayer—the most frequent "alternative treatment" used—while in a 1991 community survey of generally healthy Midwesterners, one in three reported that they had used prayer to complement their traditional medical treatments, not as a treatment substitute.[5]

Therefore, when it comes to prayer, the one-in-four number found in the Eisenberg survey ranks relatively low when compared to these surveys of patients undergoing surgery or with chronic illness or arthritis. Indeed, in one inpatient population survey, nearly 50 percent of patients desired to have their physician pray with them about their illness if the physician was comfortable doing so.[6] That half of these patients would desire such prayer shows the significance they place on it. In the face of such patient desire, several colleagues have laid out guidelines for clinicians who consider praying with their patients to address relevant boundary, competency, and ethical issues.[7]

The Use of Spiritual Healing

Turning to the published findings concerning spiritual healing, one common feature is that so little has been published in the traditional-medicine, peer-reviewed clinical research about the patient need for and use of spiritual healing. Although Benor has thoroughly summarized what is state-of-the-art in the research, these findings have received scant attention in Western medicine.[8] Exceptions include Hodges and Scofield highlighting the relevance of spiritual healing for many patients and reviewing some of the evidence from Benor. They concluded that the extent of the research was sufficient to substantiate spiritual healing as a "scientifically-attested phenomenon."[9] Others have discussed the need for more research.[10] Favazza noted the importance of spiritual healing for many patients with mental illness and the need for clinical providers to develop a greater appreciation of the cultural relevance of healing for their spiritual and religiously committed patients.[11]

As for the frequency of patient use of spiritual healing, although only a few patient surveys have looked at its use, the level of use is higher than found in the Eisenberg survey. Cassileth and colleagues in 1984 followed up on 378 cancer patients from the University of Pennsylvania, finding 71 (or 19 percent) had used spiritual healing involving "prayer, incantation, laying on of hands, and similar practices directed at cancer cure through divine intervention or exorcism of the evil represented by [the] disease."[12] Quite similar to the Gallup U.S. findings noted above, 79 percent believed that the spiritual healing had a positive effect on their general health.[13]

In a 1988 survey by Goldstein and colleagues, the researchers surveyed two physician provider groups: the American Holistic Medical Association (AHMA)—a group of alternative medicine clinicians limited to physicians and medical students—and three groups of family medicine (FM) physicians from California.[14] Their findings were quite telling. Where 45 percent of the AHMA sample felt spiritual healing had "much value for medical practice," only 9 percent of the FM sample had a similar view. In addition, 54 percent of the AHMA sample felt that spiritual healing had "some or much value and utilized it in [their] practice." In contrast, one in five, or 20 percent, of FM physicians had the same view.

The researchers also surveyed the physicians' views concerning "laying on of hands." While 20 percent of AHMA physicians felt it was of "much value for medical practice," only 3.5 percent of FM physicians held that view. Concerning whether they felt it to be of "some or much value and utilized in [their] practice," 30 percent of the AHMA sample agreed, as opposed to about 6 percent of the FM group.

The researchers looked more closely at how religious or spiritual experiences had shaped the views of the two physician samples. Mean spirituality scores for the AHMA group were twice those of the FM group. Almost half of the AHMA physicians viewed spiritual factors to be "very important" in shaping their views of health, versus one-seventh of the FM group. Interestingly, physicians from the AHMA were more likely than those from the FM to have had spiritual or religious experiences as adults (76 percent versus 40 percent) or in the last two years (32 percent versus 12 percent), or to have had "peak or transcent" experiences (72 percent versus 36 percent). While 60 percent of the AHMA physicians viewed religion or spirituality as "very important," only 18 percent of the California FM physicians felt similarly.

Findings like these reveal that, in part, it might be the influence of a provider's spirituality or religion that leads to whether they address patients' spiritual issues. Both Galanter and colleagues[15] and Olive[16] found that physicians who were more religious, whether psychiatrists or family practitioners, do pay greater attention to such factors. In the future, all practitioners, whether pro, neutral, or antispiritual, should learn to address such issues when they are found to be of substantial relevance or importance to the patient.

In a primary care physician (internal medicine and family medicine) survey by Blumberg and colleagues, the researchers asked if the physicians would: (1) encourage or discourage patient use of spiritual healing, (2) refer patients to a spiritual healer, and (3) provide spiritual healing to their patients.[17] They found about one-quarter of the physician sample would encourage and one-quarter would discourage spiritual healing "if the patient expressed interest." Interestingly, three-fourths of the physicians would be willing to refer to a spiritual healer, and 5 percent are already providing spiritual healing to their patients.

As to how frequently patients receive or practice spiritual healing, previous studies seldom assessed the rates, but those that did remained similar to Eisenberg's 4 percent, generally lower than the 5 percent found in the Blumberg study. And although the latter study found three in four physicians willing to refer if the patient so desired, in the few studies that include spiritual referral rates, they seemed to be much lower.

Finally, methodologically speaking, Eisenberg's simply quantifying the use of prayer or spiritual healing is in order given either the frequent patient use of prayer or the potential cultural relevance of spiritual healing. However, we would suggest that the best clinical research approach may not be simply counting if patients use prayer or spiritual healing but rather also how and why certain groups of patients might use or cope with such spiritual or religious practices.

Severe Illness and Spirituality

Coping with severe illness appears to encourage spirituality. For example, in a 1984 study published in *Cancer,* Eidinger and Schapira found that 34 percent of the patients had become more religious after learning of their cancer diagnosis. Among those who had become more religious, more than 50 percent prayed more frequently, 29 percent began reading or increased their reading of the Bible, and 19 percent began or increased their church attendance.[18] Similarly, in a 1997 patient survey of women with gynecologic cancer, almost half had become more religious following their cancer diagnosis. More than 90 percent felt their faith sustained their hopes, 75 percent said it had a significant place in their lives, and more than 40 percent said it enhanced their self-worth.[19] Other studies have found the importance of spiritual and religious beliefs in coping with other cancers and serious medical illnesses as well.[20]

A 1999 study on the role of religious and spiritual beliefs in coping with cancer found a significantly positive relationship between the spirituality measure and an active coping style.[21] The study's authors noted, "These findings [and others reviewed by the authors] appear to contradict the long-standing theoretical view that religious beliefs and practices represent a less than optimal means of coping with crises, in general, and with life-threatening illness, in particular. It is becoming scientifically clearer that a system of belief actually helps reduce the degree of psychological distress brought on by a life-threatening illness."[22] In other reviews of the research, researchers have similarly found that spirituality and religion were utilized as relevant "means of coping [and that these patients] seemed to deal more effectively with illness than those who do not use religious means of coping."[23]

Recognition by the American College of Physicians

With research findings like these, it is not surprising that, in a 1999 American College of Physicians-American Society of Internal Medicine Consensus Panel, the panel members recognized and highlighted the need to explore spiritual issues with patients facing end-of-life health and care. In Table 2 of their report, the panel members highlighted spiritual and religious questions that included: (1) Is faith (religion, spirituality) important to you in this illness? (2) Has faith (religion, spirituality) been important to you at other times in your life? (3) Do you have someone to talk to about religious matters? (4) Would you like to explore religious matters with someone?[24]

One (of three) tables of questions dealt directly with how clinicians can better ask patients about their faith, spirituality, or religious commitment. A consensus panel of leading clinicians underscoring the need for physicians to ask about patient faith when patients are dealing with severe medical illness is a substantial shift in clinical care.[25]

New Medical Paradigm Includes Spirituality

As seen with the American College of Physicians Consensus Panel, medical clinicians, educators, and researchers are currently undergoing a paradigm shift in which the role of spiritual factors is becoming recognized in health and mental health. The previous, more traditional medical paradigm neglected patient spiritual and religious commitment as relevant clinical factors, viewing them as too controversial, unimportant, or even as irrelevant to patients.[26] In addition, clinicians and researchers assumed spirituality was too difficult to measure, or was based on private, individual transcendent beliefs that could not be researched. Yet the impact of spiritual and religious factors can be researched. The following sections will briefly review key issues concerning (1) survey findings regarding patient need and relevance, (2) new trends in medical education to teach students how to take a spiritual history and address patients' spiritual issues, and (3) the opportunity for further research based on the historical neglect and mismeasurement of studying these factors.

The Need for Sensitivity to Patients' Religion and Spirituality

Thomas S. Kuhn's seminal work *The Structure of Scientific Revolutions* describes how the acceptance of new paradigms takes time, coming only after the old paradigm's deficiencies are accepted and demonstrated. Only after the limitations of the more transitional model are shown—often through new research—do clinicians and researchers begin to challenge the older, antiquated theory and develop a new paradigm that can better integrate the new findings or factors, as in the case of patient spirituality. New and growing research has revealed the links between religious commitment and physical and mental health in preventing illness, coping with disease and stress, and enhancing recovery, as well as living longer lives. Thus, over time medicine is beginning to develop a health care model that includes the patient's spiritual dimension.

Some clinicians remain reductionist in attributing the relationships and effects of religious commitment to "nothing but" social support or "nothing but" practicing healthier lifestyles. Yet as the research is improving and these potential mediating factors are being controlled for in studies, religious commitment still stands out as a beneficial clinical factor. An increasing number of medical researchers and practitioners are now acknowledging the relevance of religious commitment in preventing, coping with, and recovering from illness.[27]

Respecting Patient Worldviews

What can happen when patient spirituality is left out of clinical care? An example was developed by the American Psychiatric Association in 1990 in the document "Guidelines Regarding Possible Conflicts between Psychiatrists' Religious Commitments and Psychiatric Practice." The guidelines gave an illustration of a religious man treated by a psychiatrist with a differing worldview. The psychiatrist denigrated his patient's long-standing religious commitment, calling it "foolishly neurotic." The guidelines noted, "Because of the intensity of the therapeutic relationship, the interpretations caused great distress and appeared related to a subsequent suicide attempt." The guidelines underscored that instead, "[p]sychiatrists should maintain respect for their patients' beliefs."[28]

Recognizing the religious worldviews often held by the general public is a critical first step for clinicians in becoming more sensitive to this important cultural factor. For more than a half century, the Gallup Organization has polled Americans concerning their religious and spiritual beliefs. During this time, the proportion of Americans who believe in God has remained remarkably constant: 96 percent in 1944 and 95 percent in 1993. Furthermore, 85 percent of Americans consider religion "very important" or "fairly important" in their lives.[29] Nearly 40 percent attend one of the five hundred thousand places of worship in the United States weekly, including synagogues, mosques, and churches.

These trends will quite probably continue with the next generation, based on a 1992 national Gallup survey of teenagers. Large numbers of young Americans believe in God (95 percent), pray alone frequently (42 percent), read scriptures weekly (36 percent), and attend services weekly (45 percent). Somewhat surprisingly, in the early 1990s, 27 percent of teens considered religious faith more important to them than to their parents.[30]

Since, according to national survey data, religion plays a central role in many Americans' lives, do patients want spiritual issues addressed by their physicians? A 1999 University of Pennsylvania study found that a majority of patients would welcome a question from their doctors about whether they had spiritual or religious beliefs that would influence their medical decisions if they became gravely ill. In fact, 66 percent noted that their trust in the doctor would grow if asked such a question. Of those who indicated that they did have religious or spiritual beliefs that would make a difference, 94 percent felt physicians should ask. Also, as many as half of those without such beliefs thought doctors should at least inquire, the study found. In contrast, only 15 percent of the patients studied recalled having been asked whether their religious or spiritual beliefs would influence their medical decisions—a large gap between the number of those who would like to discuss it and the number of physicians who have invited them to.[31]

In a 1994 survey published in *The Journal of Family Practice,* a sample of more than two hundred inpatients found that 77 percent said physicians should consider patients' spiritual needs. Furthermore, as already noted, nearly one in two, or 48 percent, wanted their physicians to pray with them. However, about one in three, or only 32 percent, stated their physician had ever discussed their religious beliefs with them.[32] Similarly, a national poll conducted by *USA Weekend* found that 63 percent of those surveyed felt that physicians should talk to patients about their spiritual faith, but only 10 percent of their doctors had done so.[33]

Barriers to Addressing Spiritual Issues

Why have so few physicians addressed spiritual issues? Some physicians may think such issues are too complex to address. But Daaleman and Nease noted that they are not. They suggested that one way to address these issues is to use as a proxy a patient's regular or frequent religious service attendance—whether synagogue, mosque, or church—as a screen for those who view their spirituality or religion as relevant to their care.[34] In addition to a lack of awareness of clinical importance, physicians may be somewhat uncomfortable with the subject matter. Ellis and colleagues noted that the concerns primary care physicians had in addressing such issues include (1) lack of time, (2) lack of experience or skills in taking a spiritual history, (3) uncertainty about how to identify those who want to discuss spiritual issues, and (4) a concern that they would project or push their beliefs on their patients.[35]

Yet as noted by physicians Daaleman and Nease in *The Journal of Family Practice,* "Spiritual and religious issues have a place in the physician-patient encounter since they are a component of patient health and well-being."[36] These researchers also found in their study of family medicine patients that by taking a spiritual history along with a social and physical history, a physician could identify those patients who may want to address spiritual issues. As noted above, some 90 percent of patients who attended religious services monthly or more felt doctors should refer to chaplains or clergy, and 68 percent felt a religious evaluation or history should be part of the medical record.

Most primary care physicians would be sensitive to the relevance of spiritual issues, according to a survey of active members of the American Academy of Family Physicians. A quite substantial 74 percent reported attending worship service at least monthly, with nearly four in five reporting a strong religious (or spiritual) orientation and nearly 85 percent feeling somewhat or extremely close to a Higher Power or Force.[37] In addition, based on the results from the same survey, Daaleman and Frey found many physicians—more than 80 percent—referred patients to clergy or chaplains. Indeed, a quite substantial 30 percent of physicians referred more than ten patients per year to clergy or chaplains. Physicians who were more religious or who have been in practice more than fifteen years were more likely to refer to clergy or chaplains.[38]

In contrast, that many mental health professionals may lack awareness of the importance of the patient's religious beliefs or religious language could stem from diminished personal interest in religion compared to the general population. For example, according to Gallup poll data, while 6 percent of the U.S. population as a whole is atheist or agnostic, 21 percent of psychiatrists and 28 percent of clinical psychologists are atheists or agnostic. Also, while among the U.S. population more than 70 percent agreed with the statement "My whole approach to life is based on my religion," only two in five psychiatrists and one in three clinical psychologists agreed with a similar statement: "My religious faith is the most important influence in my life."[39] Many mental health professionals may be dealing with patients whose rather strong religious views differ from their own. Clinical education during medical school and the residency years can thus play a crucial role in helping these professionals begin to understand the relevance and importance of their patients' religious culture.

Many physicians may still be unaware of the importance of spiritual issues for patients as they struggle and cope with chronic or serious illness. One study at Duke University Medical Center found that 44 percent of inpatients thought that religious beliefs were the most important factor in coping with their illness, compared to only 9 percent of physicians.[40]

Why do patients so strongly perceive the potential relevance of spirituality to their medical care? A decline in physical health may precipitate a spiritual crisis. When serious illness strikes, patients often start to question their purpose in life, the meaning of their work, their relationships, and their personal identity, as well as broader meaning, life purpose, or ultimate destiny. Furthermore, patients hospitalized with severe medical illnesses face high stress, including stress or anxiety about their diagnosis, potential pain from their illness and therapeutic procedures, a sense of isolation, and a loss of control over personal activities like going to work, being with their family, eating, and sleeping.

As a result of this stress, almost one-half of hospitalized patients experience some degree of clinical depression, found Dr. Harold Koenig. In a study funded by the National Institute of Mental Health, nearly 40 percent of seriously ill patients said that religious beliefs or practices were their most important means of handling stress, and over half said they used religious coping such as prayer and scripture reading to a large extent.[41] Other studies discussed below have shown that religious coping can help prevent depression among the seriously ill, and those who do get depressed recover faster.[42] Religion can play an important role in how a patient handles stress and distress.

How does religious coping help? In his study of severely physically ill patients, Dr. Koenig found religious coping helped provide the following: (1) *strength* to cope with their condition; (2) *meaning* to help make sense of their suffering; (3) *control* over their condition because they could pray to God, who they believe is ultimately in control; (4) *hope* for a cure, hope they will be able to cope, hope for their families and loved ones, hope for life after death; and (5) *purpose, usefulness, and a sense of mission,* which help preserve self-esteem in the midst of a stressful, painful, or debilitating illness.[43]

As Foglio and Brody have noted, "The family physician who would heal cannot choose whether to confront religious variables in practice; they are operating whether recognized or not."[44] Thus, when doctors ask patients about these deeper spiritual issues, their patients may recognize the support as well as the compassion of their physicians. Not only are graduate physicians recognizing the relevance of these factors, but medical students are learning to talk with patients about their spiritual beliefs and what gives meaning to their lives.

Medical Schools Address Clinical Relevance of Spirituality

In the past, as noted above, religion was rarely mentioned in medical schools. It was deemed a topic too controversial or too personal, too nebulous, and of little clinical relevance. However, this lack of attention in medical education has shifted as a result of the impact of the growing wealth of research findings showing significant clinical importance to a great majority of patients. In the early 1990s, only two or three medical schools offered courses on spirituality. By 1999, some sixty-two medical schools were incorporating instruction in how to address patients' spiritual concerns, with twenty-seven having received John Templeton Foundation Awards, including Johns Hopkins, Harvard, Georgetown, Brown, Emory, Vanderbilt, and George Washington. Starting in 1995, the Templeton Foundation Awards have been given to medical school courses of excellence in spirituality and medicine. The awards have been given annually, and winners are determined through a national competitive review process. The patient surveys as well as the clinical research findings, along with recognition of ethical and sensitive ways to address this factor to facilitate patients' coping and recovery, have opened up course after course.

Key components in the medical school courses have been developed over time by the individual medical schools. These course components include (1) teaching students to include a spiritual evaluation or assessment as part of routine history in a respectful, nonjudgmental, and nonimposing fashion; (2) reviewing published research on the role of spirituality and health; (3) cooperating with chaplains and other spiritual counselors as integral members of the health care team; and (4) reviewing major religious traditions and specific clinical relationships of these traditions that may influence or affect health care choices and patient coping.[45]

Beneficial Research Findings

Since what is taught in medical schools should be supported by published research, the question of adding a new factor, potentially controversial in medicine, such as spirituality, must also be investigated. Not only are these research studies relevant in training the next generation of physicians, but more importantly they are relevant for more sensitively improving the care and outcomes for patients, particularly for those with severe and chronic illness.

Empirical evidence for the link between spirituality and health is currently mounting in studies published in peer-reviewed medical journals. Published studies are finding that religious and spiritual commitment is linked with improved recovery from surgery, better coping with severe medical illness and major depression, reduced hospital stays, lower blood pressure, longer life, suicide prevention, and prevention and treatment of substance abuse.

In 1998, the collaboration of more than seventy top researchers in the fields of physical and mental health, addictions, and the neurosciences culminated in a consensus report to review current research findings and to map out future research directions as well as barriers to overcome. The consensus report stated: "The data from many of the studies conducted to date are both sufficiently robust and tantalizing to warrant continued and expanded clinical investigations."[46] A comprehensive review of more than one thousand studies can be found in the publication titled *Handbook of Religion and Health*.[47] Unfortunately, the scope of this chapter prevents us from reviewing these many published studies here.

The Need for a Solid Research Base on Spirituality and Health

Despite benefits found in many individual studies of published research, most clinical fields have continued to overlook researching religious/spiritual factors. Studies with these variables are often missing in the field's best journals. In an editorial published in *The Journal of Family Practice,* ethicists Jacob Foglio and Howard Brody highlighted the need for better research on patient spirituality and religion in medicine. Commenting on the importance of conducting empirical studies, these authors stated:

> Research into religious issues and variables in family medicine might be rejected or undervalued because it seems wedded to the realm of anecdote or opinion. Ironically, the absence of a solid literature on religion and family medicine will assure that our knowledge remains in the realm of anecdote and opinion, instead of progressing to the empirical assessment of beneficial, neutral, and harmful roles of religion among patients and providers.[48]

Researchers have shown that Foglio and Brody remain quite correct in noting substantial deficits not only in family medicine in measuring spiritual and religious factors but in other relevant clinical fields as well. Replicable "systematic reviews" of the published research show a scarcity of research, lagging behind the changes in medical education and mounting clinical awareness of the importance of religious/spirituals factors for patients in their coping with serious illness.

The Systematic Review

To assess how often as well as how well fields have included religious commitment variables, we undertook the systematic reviews described below. The systematic review method owes its conceptualization to work by Richard Light and David Pillemer in their book *Summing Up*.[49] By using an objective review method, the systematic review minimizes the opportunity for reviewer bias found in the more usual and more traditional review approach. In addition, systematic reviews are quite specific in terms of the kinds of studies and study populations that are to be reviewed or assessed.

The sampling frame for the systematic review most frequently comprises all quantified articles in certain leading journals published during a certain number of years. The systematic review does not review case reports, commentaries, or editorials. Variables of interest to be reviewed are specified and identified, such as various quantified measures of religious commitment. The review team then searches by hand through every article within the specified sampling frame to identify articles containing any of the variables under review. Running totals are kept on the number of articles scanned and the number of articles and measures contained on the topic of interest. Also specified are the methods for analyzing the quality of the studies, determining and specifying interrater reliability (generally above 0.80), and summing the results across the reviewed studies. Results can be simply presented and understood as numeric items, and the review findings and results, like any good research protocol, can be replicated. In summary, the systematic review objectively assesses the quantity and quality of studies in a particular research area or field.

A Systematic Review of Psychiatry Journals

Our first such review concerned psychiatry's research handling of spiritual and religious factors in its leading journals.[50] We reviewed the *American Journal of Psychiatry, British Journal of Psychiatry, Canadian Journal of Psychiatry,* and the *Archives of General Psychiatry* from 1978 through 1982. We sought to discover how often and how well the quantified research studies contained a quantified religious variable, or religious variables about which data were collected. For instance, a religious commitment variable might be a response to a question asking how important was one's spirituality or how frequently a person prays or attends religious worship services.

During the five-year period in those four journals, 3,777 articles were published, 2,348 of which included quantitative data. Among the quantitative studies, only 59, or 2.5 percent, included one or more religious measures. Significantly, in only 3 of the 2,348 studies was a religious variable a central focus of the study. In addition, we found that less than 1 percent of all quantitative studies published in these major psychiatric journals included a methodologically acceptable religious commitment variable. Of the 59 studies that included a religious variable, most (or about 63 percent) measured religious commitment with denomination as the quantified variable, usually an irrelevant clinical measure since it does not reveal level of spiritual practices or importance of beliefs. As for the number of religious measures used, most (83 percent) of these 59 studies used a single question, although neither spiritual nor religious commitment is best studied with a "single-item" measurement approach. Only one study out of the 2,348 quantitative studies included the state-of-the-art, a multidimensional religious commitment questionnaire employing an array of items that had earlier been statistically tested to assess the measure's reliability. This systematic review revealed how infrequently and how inadequately psychiatry studied spiritual or religious commitment in its research literature.

Was Spirituality Clinically Harmful or Beneficial in Psychiatry Journals?

Given these initial review results, we took a step further and asked if religion was as harmful as psychiatry had historically assumed. To answer this question, we conducted a systematic review of the two leading American psychiatry journals from 1978 to 1989 to see if the association with mental health was beneficial, negative, or neutral.[51] We hypothesized the results to be a bell-shaped curve, with preponderant neutral findings with a few harmful and a few positive findings as well.

All quantified religious measures were located in the studies published in the *American Journal of Psychiatry* and the *Archives of General*

Psychiatry during those years. The review of all relevant studies published during the twelve years in these two leading journals of psychiatry found 139 religious commitment measures employed in the quantitative studies. Somewhat surprisingly, for only 50 (36 percent) of the 139 measures did the studies actually report an association between religious commitment and mental health. No findings were presented for the 89 other studies, meaning that for the majority, data either remained unanalyzed or were analyzed and not reported. Among the 50 results reported, the findings revealed that 72 percent were positive associations with mental health, 16 percent were negative, and 12 percent were nonsignificant. This differed widely from the bell-shaped curve with primarily neutral associations that we had hypothesized. In fact, some 92 percent of four out of the six relevant spiritual or religious dimensions were beneficial to mental health status: (1) participating in religious ceremony, (2) religion as social support, (3) prayer, and (4) relationship with God. These results were substantially more positive than what was formally or informally taught at that time in most psychiatry residency programs regarding religion and mental health.

Finally, and quite surprisingly, in most studies where a religious commitment variable was specified, no hypothesis was given. Only 30 (22 percent) of the 139 measures presented a research hypothesis. This important and quite critical research deficit showed the need for psychiatry to become far more intentional about its methods and approach in studying religion and spirituality.

Systematic Reviews of Other Clinical Fields

In addition to psychiatry, researchers have conducted systematic reviews in other clinical fields to assess how frequently and how well religious commitment has been addressed to date, including family medicine, adolescence, mental health nursing, and psychology.

The field of family medicine often considers health and illness not only within physical, social, and emotional contexts, but spiritual as well. In order to see how often and how well religious variables were considered, a research team undertook a systematic review of all articles published in the *Journal of Family Practice* from 1976 to 1986. A total of 1,086 studies were systematically reviewed and only 3.5 percent of the articles contained a quantified religious variable—only 1 percent higher than psychiatry. Some 603 (or 55 percent) measured at least one quantified variable of any type, and 468 of those measured at least one psychosocial variable. Of the 468, only 21 studies measured at least one religious variable. In contrast to psychiatry, family medicine did employ religious commitment measures (as opposed to only denominational measures) most of the time, in about 60 percent of the studies. Yet, as with psychiatry, in only one case did it use state-of-the-art, pretested, multidimensional measures of religion.[52]

As in the case of psychiatry, the systematic review research team then analyzed these studies to see if religious commitment was found to be harmful, neutral, or beneficial to health status. Results implying a beneficial link between spiritual commitment and health were almost three times as frequent as the results showing harmful relationships. Somewhat similar to the psychiatry review, the dimensions of social support, ceremony, and relationship with God were positive in twenty-one cases and neutral in three, with no negative effects exhibited. Denomination's sixteen results showed no effect, not surprising since denomination is a demographic simply acknowledging one's affiliation, not really measuring levels of spiritual or religious commitment. "Meaning" references had high levels of negative associations—about half. Similarly, for the category "unclear," four out of six associations were also negative. The results for "unclear" are not surprising, since for the "unclears" the reviewers were not certain exactly what the study variable was measuring.[53]

Like the first systematic review, this review found that the field of family medicine had a long way to go in improving research methodology to include reliable religious commitment measures more frequently. Nevertheless, as in psychiatry, when religious commitment measures were included, albeit very simple in their single-item approach, the studies found generally positive links with health status.

How does the field of adolescence research stand in recognizing the clinical relevance of religious commitment? Are there certain at-risk behaviors where greater research attention to religious commitment could reduce risk or enhance care? A systematic review of quantitative studies published in five leading adolescent journals between 1992 and 1996 revealed that 109, or nearly 12 percent, out of 922 articles included a measure of religious commitment. When compared with psychiatry and family medicine, this more than fourfold increase suggests that adolescence researchers are more sensitive to the role of religious factors. Furthermore, regarding quality, in almost half the studies investigating religion, two or more measures of religious commitment were used, as opposed to only a single measure. These systematic review findings indicate adolescent studies also tend to have improved method-ological designs.[54] Thus, adolescent researchers are recognizing religion and spirituality as relevant factors in their research to a greater degree than in either psychiatry or family medicine. Research further indicates that religious commitment can help teens reduce "at-risk" behaviors such as alcohol and drug use, delinquency, premature sexual involve-ment, unsafe sexual behaviors, and suicide.[55]

Similar to adolescence journals, a systematic review of quantitative studies in three mental health nursing journals from 1991 to 1995 found that about 10 percent—or 31 of 311 studies—included a measure of religious commitment, once again substantially higher than in psychiatry or family medicine journals. Also, almost 40 percent of these used two or more questions to assess religious commitment, as in the adolescent research, a step ahead in measurement compared to psychiatry and family medicine.[56] Nursing has a history of recognizing and affirming the importance of religion and spirituality that stands in marked contrast to the negative attitudes toward religion previously asserted by psychiatry and psychology. One of the pioneers and founders of nursing, Florence Nightingale, taught that spirituality was an integral part of human experience and compatible with scientific inquiry.[57] Furthermore, since 1988 "spiritual distress" has been an official nursing diagnosis. In addition, nurses have been much more likely to receive training in spiritual-religious issues than other mental health professionals. In a 1990 national sample, 60 percent of registered nurses said spiritual care issues had been addressed to some degree in their training. In comparison, two 1990 mental health professional surveys found that only 5 percent of psychologists had spiritual issues addressed in their training and only 18 percent of psychiatrists had received such training during their residencies.

According to a recent review of psychology, psychiatry and psychol-ogy are not very dissimilar in their infrequent research handling of spiritual and religious issues. A systematic review of seven major Ameri-can Psychological Association journals from 1991 to 1994 found that only 2.7 percent (similar to the 2.5 percent found in psychiatry)—or 62 out of 2,302 quantitative studies—contain a religious variable. In most cases—about 80 percent—measures consisted of only a single religious question. These findings suggest that psychology, again similar to psychiatry, lacks a sufficiently substantial research base to enable an adequate evaluation of the relevant, or the beneficial or harmful, effects of client religion.[58]

It should be highlighted that in the 1992 Centennial Address before the American Psychological Association, the distinguished Yale University psychologist Seymour B. Sarason lamented the absence of "transcendence" in modern psychology. He presented what he observed as a negative prejudgment of religion among many of his peers:

> I think I am safe in assuming that the bulk of the membership of the American Psychological Association would, if asked, describe themselves as agnostic or atheistic. I am also safe in assuming that any one or all of the ingredients of the religious worldview are of neither personal nor professional interest to most psychologists. And there are more than a few psychologists who not only have difficulty identifying with any of those ingredients but who also regard adherence to any of them as a reflection of irrationality, of superstition, of immaturity, of neurosis. Indeed, if we learn that someone is devoutly religious, or even tends in that direction, we look upon that person with puzzlement, often concluding that that psychologist obviously had or has personal problems.[59]

Further empirical research could better inform psychology's more traditional, nonresearch-based assumptions. The very low rate of original research that considers a religious variable within mainstream psychology remains inconsistent with the historical leadership psychology researchers have offered to the social sciences in sensitively considering client-relevant, valued personal or social influences. As a result, substantial, important opportunities remain for the field to remedy this deficiency and begin to expand and investigate the link between spirituality and mental health.

Conclusion

Patient survey data have revealed that a majority of patients desire to have their spiritual/religious framework addressed in their medical care, particularly when coping with severe illness. Some 66 percent noted that their trust in their physician would grow if asked questions regarding their spiritual/religious values. Research findings have found religious/spiritual commitment can enhance coping, help recovery from surgery, lower blood pressure, reduce depression, enhance immune system functioning, and, according to recent mortality studies, reduce the risk of earlier death by 25 percent[60] and lengthen lives by seven to fourteen years.[61]

Recognizing patient desire along with potential health benefits, more than half of U.S. medical schools now offer courses on spirituality and medicine, many of these required. The American Association of Medical Colleges will soon provide curriculum objectives that underscore the importance of addressing patients' spiritual needs as part of becoming a competent, compassionate doctor.[62] Similarly, the American College of Physicians–American Society of Internal Medicine consensus panel on end-of-life care also recommends that physicians address patient's spiritual and religious issues.

Although the body of well-designed research studies investigating links between spiritual/religious commitment continues to grow, many clinical fields have given scant attention to these factors. Opportunities await to respond to the deficits in these fields by expanding the scope of clinical research and focusing on the role of patient spirituality in clinical education and care.

NOTES

1. David M. Eisenberg et al. "Unconventional Medicine in the United States: Prevalence, Costs, and Patterns of Use," *NEJM* 328, no. 4 (1993): 246–52.

2. "GO LIFE Survey on Prayer" (Princeton: Gallup Organization, 1993).

3. Michael E. McCullough and David B. Larson, "Prayer," in *Integrating Spirituality into Treatment: Resources for Practitioners,* ed. William R. Miller (Washington, D.C.: American Psychological Association Press, 1999), pp. 85–110.

4. George Fitchett, Laurel Arthur Burton, and Abigail B. Sivan, "The Religious Needs and Resources of Psychiatric Inpatients," *Journal of Nervous and Mental Disease* 185, no. 5 (1997): 20–326; T. L. Saudia, "Health Locus of Control and Helpfulness of Prayer," *Heart and Lung* 20, no. 1 (January 1991): 60–65.

5. Judith Horstman, "The Dangerous Divide," *Arthritis Today* 13, no. 6 (1999): 35–41; Kathy K. Trier and Anson Shupe, "Prayer, Religiosity, and Healing in the Heartland, USA: A Research Note," *Review of Religious Research* 32, no. 4 (1991): 351–58.

6. Dana E. King and B. Bushwick, "Beliefs and Attitudes of Hospital Patients about Faith Healing and Prayer," *Journal of Family Medicine* 39, no. 4 (October 1994): 349–52.

7. McCullough and Larson, "Prayer"; Stephen G. Post, Christina M. Puchalski, and David B. Larson, "Physicians and Patient Spirituality: Professional Boundaries, Competency and Ethics," *Annals of Internal Medicine* 132, no. 7 (April 4, 2000): 578–83.

8. Daniel J. Benor, *Healing Research: Holistic Energy Medicine and Spirituality,* vol. 1, Research in Healing (Deddington, England: Helix Editions, 1993);

Daniel J. Benor, *Healing Research: Holistic Energy Medicine and Spirituality*, vol. 3, Research in Spiritual Healing (Deddington, England: Helix Editions, 1993).

9. R. D. Hodges and A. M. Scofield, "Is Spiritual Healing a Valid and Effective Therapy?" *Journal of the Royal Society of Medicine* 88 (April 1995): 203–07.

10. Edwin Martin, "Divine Healing: The Christian View," *Journal of the Royal College of General Practitioners* 36 (January 1986): 3; Rex Gardner, "Miracles of Healing in Anglo-Celtic Northumbria as Recorded by the Venerable Bede and His Contemporaries: A Reappraisal in the Light of Twentieth Century Experience," *British Medical Journal* 287 (December 24–31, 1983): 1927–33.

11. Armando R. Favazza, "Modern Christian Healing of Mental Illness," *American Journal of Psychiatry* 139, no. 6 (1982): 728–34.

12. Barrie R. Cassileth et al., "Contemporary Unorthodox Treatments in Cancer Medicine," *Annals of Internal Medicine* 101, no. 1 (1984): 105–12.

13. Cassileth, "Contemporary Unorthodox Treatments in Cancer Medicine."

14. Michael S. Goldstein et al., "Holistic Physicians and Family Practitioners: Similarities, Differences and Implications for Health Policy," *Social Science Medicine* 26, no. 8 (1988): 853–61.

15. Marc Galanter, David Larson, and Elizabeth Rubenstone, "Christian Psychiatry: The Impact of Evangelical Belief on Clinical Practice," *American Journal of Psychiatry* 148, no. 1 (1991): 90–95.

16. Kenneth E. Olive, "Physician Religious Beliefs and the Physician-Patient Relationship: A Study of Devout Physicians," *Southern Medical Journal* 88, no. 12 (1995): 1249–55.

17. Daniel L. Blumberg et al., "The Physician and Unconventional Medicine," *Alternative Therapies* 1, no. 3 (1995): 31–35.

18. Richard N. Eidinger and David V. Schapira, "Cancer Patients' Insight into Their Treatment, Prognosis, and Unconventional Therapies," *Cancer* 53, no. 12 (1984): 2736–40.

19. James A. Roberts et al., "Factors Influencing Views of Patients with Gynecologic Cancer about End-of-Life Decisions," *American Journal of Obstetrics and Gynecology* 176, no. 1 (January 1997): 166–72.

20. Marc A. Musick et al., "Religion, Spiritual Beliefs, and Cancer" *Psycho-Oncology,* ed. J. Holland (New York: Oxford University Press, 1998) pp. 780–89.

21. Lea Baider et al., "The Role of Religious and Spiritual Beliefs in Coping with Malignant Melanoma: An Israeli Sample," *Psycho-Oncology* 8 (1999): 27–35.

22. Baider, "The Role of Religious and Spiritual Beliefs," p. 33.

23. Dale A. Matthews et al., "Religious Commitment and Health Status," *Archives of Family Medicine* 7 (1998): 118–24, at 122.

24. Bernard Lo, Timothy Quill, and James Tulsky, "Discussing Palliative Care with Patients," *Annals of Internal Medicine* 130 (1999): 744–49.

25. Lo, Quill, and Tulsky, "Discussing Palliative Care with Patients," pp. 744–49.

26. David B. Larson and Mary G. Milano, "Making the Case for Spiritual Interventions in Clinical Practice," *Mind / Body Medicine* 2, no. 1 (1997): 20–30.

27. Matthews et al., "Religious Commitment and Health Status," pp. 118–24.

28. American Psychiatric Association Board of Trustees, "Guidelines Regarding Possible Conflict between Psychiatrists' Religious Commitment and Psychiatric Practice," *American Journal of Psychiatry* 147, no. 4 (1990): 542.

29. George H. Gallup, *Religion in America: 1992–1993* (Princeton: The Gallup Organization, 1993).

30. George H. Gallup and R. Bezilla, *The Religious Life of Young Americans* (Princeton: George Gallup International Institute, 1992).

31. John W. Ehman et al., "Do Patients Want Physicians to Inquire about Their Spiritual or Religious Beliefs If They Become Gravely Ill?" *Archives of Internal Medicine* 139 (August 9/23, 1999): 1803–06.

32. Dana E. King and B. Bushwick, "Beliefs and Attitudes of Hospital Inpatients about Faith, Healing, and Prayer," *Journal of Family Practice* 39, no. 4 (October 1994): 349–52.

33. Tom McNichol, "The New Faith in Medicine," *USA Weekend,* April 5–7, 1997, pp. 4–5.

34. Timothy P. Daaleman and Donald E. Nease, "Patient Attitudes Regarding Physician Inquiry into Spiritual and Religious Issues," *Journal of Family Practice* 39, no. 6 (1994): 564–68.

35. Mark R. Ellis, Daniel C. Vinson, and Bernard Ewigman, "Addressing Spiritual Concerns of Patients: Family Physicians' Attitudes and Practices," *Journal of Family Practice* 48, no. 2 (1999): 105–09.

36. Daaleman and Nease, "Patient Attitudes Regarding Physician Inquiry into Spiritual and Religious Issues," pp. 564–68.

37. Timothy P. Daaleman and Bruce Frey, "Spiritual and Religious Beliefs and Practices of Family Physicians: A National Survey," *Journal of Family Practice* 48, no. 2 (1999): 98–104.

38. Timothy P. Daaleman and Bruce Frey, "Prevalence and Patterns of Physician Referral to Clergy and Pastoral Care Providers," *Archives of Family Medicine* 7 (November/December 1998): 548–53.

39. Allen E. Bergin and Jay P. Jensen, "Religiosity of Psychotherapists: A National Survey," *Psychotherapy* 27, no. 1 (1990): 3–7.

40. Harold G. Koenig et al., "Religious Perspectives of Doctors, Nurses, Patients and Families," *Journal of Pastoral Care* 45 (1991): 254–67.

41. Harold G. Koenig, "Use of Religion by Patients with Severe Medical Illness," *Mind / Body Medicine* 2, no. 1 (1997): 31-43.

42. Harold G. Koenig, Linda K. George, and Bercedis L. Peterson, "Religiosity and Remission of Depression in Medically Ill Older Patients," *American Journal of Psychiatry* 155, no. 4 (1998): 536–42.

43. Koenig, "Use of Religion by Patients with Severe Medical Illness," pp. 31–43.

44. Jacob R. Foglio and Howard Brody, "Religion, Faith, and Medicine," *Journal of Family Practice* 27, no. 5 (1988): 473–74.

45. Christina M. Puchalski and David B. Larson, "Developing Curricula in Spirituality and Medicine," *Academic Medicine* 73, no. 9 (1998): 970–74.

46. David B. Larson, James P. Swyers, and Michael E. McCullough, eds., *Scientific Research on Spirituality and Health: A Consensus Report* (Rockville, Md.: National Institute for Healthcare Research, 1998).

47. Harold G. Koenig, Michael E. McCullough, and David B. Larson, *Handbook of Religion and Health* (New York: Oxford University Press, 2001).

48. Foglio and Brody, "Religion, Faith, and Medicine," p. 473.

49. Richard J. Light and David B. Pillemer, *Summing Up: The Science of Reviewing Research* (Cambridge, Mass.: Harvard University Press, 1984).

50. David B. Larson et al., "Systematic Analysis of Research on Religious Variables in Four Major Psychiatric Journals, 1978–1982," *American Journal of Psychiatry*, 149, no. 3 (March 1986): 329–34.

51. David B. Larson et al., "Dimensions and Valences of Measures of Religious Commitment Found in the American Journal of Psychiatry and the Archives of General Psychiatry: 1978 through 1989," *American Journal of Psychiatry* 149, no. 4 (April 1992): 557–59.

52. Frederick C. Craigie et al., "A Systematic Analysis of Religious Variables in *Journal of Family Practice, 1976–1986,*" *Journal of Family Practice* 27, no. 5 (1988): 509–13.

53. Frederick C. Craigie, David B. Larson, and Ingrid Y. Liu, "References to Religion in The Journal of Family Practice: Dimensions and Valence of Spirituality," *Journal of Family Practice* 30, no. 4 (1990): 477–80.

54. Andrew J. Weaver et al., "An Analysis of Research on Religious Variables in Five Major Adolescent Research Journals: 1992–1996," *Journal of Nervous and Mental Disease* 188, no. 1 (2000): 36–44.

55. John Wallace and Tyrone Forman, "Religion's Role in Promoting Health and Reducing Risk among American Youth," *Health Education and Behavior* 25, no. 6 (1998): 721–41.

56. Andrew J. Weaver et al., "An Analysis of Research on Religious and Spiritual Variables in Three Mental Health Nursing Journals, 1991–1995," *Issues in Mental Health Nursing* 19 (1998): 263–76.

57. J. Macrae, "Nightingale's Spiritual Philosophy and Its Significance for Modern Nursing," *Image: Journal of Nursing Scholarship* 27, no. 1 (1995): 8–10.

58. Andrew J. Weaver et al., "Is Religion Taboo in Psychology? A Systematic Analysis of Research on Religious Variables in Seven Major American Psychological Association Journals: 1991–1994," *Journal of Psychology and Christianity* 17, no. 3 (1998): 220–32.

59. S. B. Sarason, "American Psychology and the Need for Transcendence and Community," *American Journal of Community Psychology* 21 (1993): 185–202.

60. William J. Strawbridge et al., "Frequent Attendance at Religious Services and Mortality over 28 Years," *American Journal of Public Health* 87, no. 6 (1997): 957–61.

61. Robert A. Hummer et al., "Religious Involvement and U.S. Adult Mortality," *Demography* 36, no. 2 (1999): 1–13.

62. *Report III Contemporary Issues in Medicine: Communication in Medicine, Medical School Objectives Project* (Washington, D.C.: Association of American Medical Colleges, October 1999), pp. 1–28.

ASBJØRN HRÓBJARTSSON AND STIG BRORSON

Interpreting Results from Randomized Clinical Trials of Complementary/ Alternative Interventions: The Role of Trial Quality and Pre-trial Beliefs

In 1997, approximately four out of ten American citizens used complementary/alternative interventions, and the expenditures on such therapies were conservatively estimated to be $27 billion.[1] Complementary/ alternative medicine as a social phenomenon is an important subject for medical humanities and the social sciences, regardless of whether these interventions in general are associated with therapeutic effects. However, from the point of view of practical consumers, funding health authorities, and clinical science, the question of therapeutic effect is paramount.

The randomized trial is generally regarded to be the gold standard in evaluating effects of health interventions.[2] The role of randomized trials in complementary/alternative medicine has been debated, but the number of complementary/alternative randomized trials actually conducted is remarkably high.[3] For example, in 1999 the Cochrane Library listed more than four thousand controlled trials of complementary/alternative interventions, while a further four thousand awaited assessment.[4]

This chapter provides a general discussion of the interpretation of results from randomized trials of complementary/alternative interventions. First, we focus on the methodological quality of the design and conduct of the trial; second, we discuss the role played by pre-trial beliefs. We shall argue that, when appraising clinical trials of complementary/ alternative interventions, it is reasonable to interpret results cautiously when trials have design inadequacies and when the interventions are based on theories regarded as scientifically implausible.

It is difficult to characterize complementary/alternative interventions, as the various therapies that currently fall under that name differ greatly in theoretical background and in the interventions practiced. We often refer to homeopathy in our discussion because it is an interesting case for two reasons: (1) it is easily tested in randomized double-blind trials, and (2) the plausibility of the background theory is very low from a standard scientific point of view.

Bias in Complementary/Alternative Trials

Positive results in clinical trials are reflections of either chance findings, the effect of the interventions, or bias. The risk of a chance finding is addressed with appropriate statistical analysis and will be discussed later. The possibility of bias requires a critical evaluation of the design and conduct of the trial. Below, we will first present some selected empirical studies that find exaggerated effects in clinical trials with inadequate methodological design. Then we will discuss the general methodological quality of complementary/alternative trials.

Empirical Evidence of Bias in Randomized Trials of Mainstream Medicine

Several empirical studies have been conducted with the purpose of identifying dimensions of randomized trials that are associated with exaggerated effects.[5] Schulz and colleagues demonstrated that in obstetrical and neonatal trials with binary outcomes, odds ratios were inflated by 41 percent in the trials where randomization was conducted unconcealed, thus making it possible for participants to predict which treatment a patient would receive before formal inclusion in the trial.[6] They also found that odds ratios were exaggerated by 17 percent in trials where double-blinding was lacking. Moher studied a broad group of trials with binary, mostly objective outcomes and found similar bias in trials with unconcealed allocation, but no bias in trials that lacked double-blinding.[7]

The studies referred to above differ considerably in overall design, types of included trials, outcomes, and other setting factors. Thus, the association between the magnitude of the bias and the design factor studied—for example, randomization or double-blinding—can be true for the specific group of trials included in the study, but one should be cautious in extrapolating the exact numerical findings to all trials, including to complementary/alternative trials. For example, it cannot be ignored that double-blinding could be just as important as randomization in trials with "soft outcomes," such as patients' or evaluators' reports of overall improvement.

The Quality of Randomized Trials of Complementary/ Alternative Interventions

Several reviews have assessed the methodology of complementary/ alternative trials and reported a general low quality. One review identified more than five thousand complementary/alternative trials and registered how many trials met four basic requirements, including that randomization was described and that either observer or patients (or both) were blinded. Only 258 trials met these criteria. Approximately 90 percent of the exclusions were due to lack of randomization or blinding. The included trials were further analyzed for methodological quality according to a scoring system, and the authors concluded that "the quality of the evaluated studies was low."[8] Similar conclusions were reported in systematic reviews of randomized trials of acupuncture for chronic pain and of homeopathy trials.[9]

The general low quality in trials of complementary/alternative intervention raises the suspicion of bias. We have not been able to find studies that directly investigate the association between low trial quality and exaggerated effects in a broad population of complementary/alternative trials, however the systematic review of homeopathy trials referred to above indicates a clear association between low trial quality and exaggerated effects.[10] The combined odds ratio for eighty-nine randomized or double-blind trials comparing homeopathy with placebo was 2.45, a result that strongly favors homeopathy. The combined odds ratio of the twenty-six trials scoring high on two quality scales was clearly lower, 1.66, but still statistically significant. There has been a heated scientific debate about how to interpret this result.[11] Some have concluded that it is now proven that homeopathy works. Others have been more cautious, including the authors of the original review. When quality was assessed without using formal quality scales, the authors considered that only 10 percent (or approximately nine trials) were actually of high quality, but they did not report the combined odds ratio. In a follow-up article, they identified lack of double blinding as an especially important source of bias, and on the basis of several rigorous trials conducted after the review was published they concluded that "it seems likely that our meta-analysis at least overestimated the effects of homeopathic treatments."[12] In the present discussion of bias we are not concerned with whether the odds ratio of 1.66 was biased or not; however, the overall result of 2.45 was clearly exaggerated due to low-quality trials.

The bias found in the homeopathy trials is remarkable also because the trials were double-blinded or randomized (only eight trials were not double-blinded). Thus the substantial bias must be explained by factors other than lack of blinding and randomization. One possibility is that the sample of trials included in the review was unrepresentative and negative trials were missing. Journals tend to publish small positive trials quicker and more often than small negative trials—the so-called publication bias. However, we find it unlikely that publication bias is the full explanation. When it comes to homeopathy and complementary/alternative medicine, it could be the case that standard medical journals would prefer to publish negative results.

There are numerous possible design inadequacies that could explain the bias found. However, in many cases these will reflect specific problems related to the participants included in the trial, the intervention they received, the control group, and the outcome. Our aim is to discuss bias more generally in complementary/alternative randomized trials. Thus, instead of a systematic presentation of the possible sources of bias, we focus on two background factors that we find relevant not only for trials of homeopathy, but for complementary/alternative trials in general: logistics and conflicts of interest.

Logistics

Quality analyses of randomized trials are often based on analyses of trial reports and not of the conduct of the trial. This can be problematic, as important aspects of methodology may not be described or important problematic points may be omitted. Furthermore, when central dimensions of trial methodology are evaluated in a trial report, an unproblematic relationship between the trial investigators' intention and the actual execution of the trial is often assumed. However, the randomized trial is a fragile research instrument. It is basically a social enterprise in which the real content of design features, for example randomization and double-blinding, depend on the practical implementation of a complex infrastructure. Therefore, the risk of bias does not only depend on the intended design but on how rigorously the practical trial execution was carried out and how efficient control measures were in preventing protocol violations or detecting insignificant protocol violations before they became serious. For example, there are numerous examples of double-blind trials from mainstream medicine in which the double-blinding was broken.[13]

The big logistical challenges in the practical conduct of randomized trials have resulted in the development of guidelines for monitoring clinical investigations, the so-called standards of good clinical (research) practice, often implying a process of auditing.[14] To conduct a trial according to the standards of good clinical research practice is the norm in many biomedical pharmacological trials. We have not been able to find any existing study of how many homeopathy trials, or other complementary/alternative trials, have been conducted according to standards of good clinical practice.

It seems prudent to suspect bias in trials conducted with inadequate logistical support. It is an interesting question whether complementary/alternative trials in general have fewer resources, people, experienced leading trial investigators, and auditing procedures than mainstream medicine trials.

Conflicts of Interest

It is generally accepted that the risk of bias is higher than usual when a trial is conducted by investigators with a strong interest in a special result. This has led most leading medical journals to ask contributors to declare any conflict of interest, thus complying with the statements of the fifth edition of the uniform requirements for manuscripts submitted to biomedical journals by the International Committee of Medical Journal Editors (the so-called Vancouver Group).[15] There are good reasons for this practice. Examples of the influence of commercial interests on the conclusions of scientific papers can be found in research on the effects of tobacco. As many as twenty-seven out of fifty-six primary studies funded by the tobacco industry concluded that nicotine enhanced cognitive functions, but when studies were not funded by the tobacco industry, sixteen out of seventeen studies concluded that no such effect could be found.[16]

Commercial interests are not confined to mainstream medicine. For example, homeopathic preparations and various herbal medicines are produced for profit, and there is little reason to believe that complementary/alternative trials are immune to economic bias. For example, in a trial of the effect of Ginseng on quality of life scores, the second author was a senior employee of the pharmaceutical company producing the Ginseng product.[17] The result of the trial was positive, but possibly biased due to differential dropout in the two compared groups.

It is interesting that, in statements of "the uniform requirements for manuscripts" referred to above, conflicts of interests are not only economic but also "academic competition, and intellectual passion." The passion of the trial investigators and the competing environment of the research are not emphasized in handbooks on research methodology. However, such factors are essential when discussing complementary/ alternative medicine, as the disagreements between the medical "sceptics" and the alternative "believers" are often heated and reveal both strong passions and competition.

It is essential for a reliable trial result that investigators be genuinely interested in finding out whether the intervention tested works or not. If the trial investigators are all strong believers, this may induce bias, due for example, to lack of appropriate data handling, insufficient rigor in trial execution, or even direct fraud. Similarly, if all trial investigators are strong sceptics, the bias can be negative. In other words, the basic loyalty of the investigators must be to the scientific question and method and not to the intervention tested or to any competing intervention.

It is difficult, if not impossible, to assess such an abstract entity as loyalty to a scientific question and method. However, within mainstream medicine this loyalty at times comes under pressure, for example through strong feelings for a promising new treatment, fatigue about the logistical rigor of the trial execution, and the need for career promoting publications. Similarly, the loyalty of some complementary/alternative trial investigators to the scientific question and method may also be strained. Many complementary/alternative practitioners have no thorough scientific training and generally have strong feelings for their interventions. Furthermore, complementary/alternative medicine sometimes represents not only a class of interventions, but also an existential position in which the interventions practised are intimately linked to semireligious metaphysical positions. It is a controversial question whether complementary/alternative trial investigators in general are less loyal to the scientific question and method than trial investigators in mainstream medicine.

Pre-trial Beliefs

When evaluating whether an apparent effect in a randomized trial reflects a true effect, probability considerations are involved on two levels. First, even the most thorough analysis of methodological trial quality can only conclude that there are or are not overt signs of bias, but it can never exclude hidden bias, for example due to unregistered protocol violations. The decision to trust the result in a given trial is based on a personal belief that the likelihood of bias is low. The second level of probability considerations is the evaluation of possible chance findings in a clinical trial. In the following section, we will address these considerations, focusing on the role played by pre-trial beliefs. We find it fruitful to conceptualize this issue within the frame of Bayesian reasoning.

The Bayesian Perspective

Within evidence-based medicine, evaluations of and choices between clinical interventions are, by definition, based on evidence. However, the world faced by clinical researchers is not a world exclusively constituted of crude facts ready to be discovered. The interpretation of new evidence always depends, to a certain degree, on what is already known; that is, on old evidence. Within medical epidemiology and philosophy, this view is usually termed "the Bayesian perspective." According to this perspective, observers evaluate new evidence in light of their background knowledge. In the evaluation process, an estimated probability that a given event will occur, often called "the prior probability," cannot be neglected when interpreting new evidence. On the basis of both the prior probability and the new evidence, "posterior probability" is determined. Consequently, if prior probability is estimated to be low, a considerable amount of positive evidence is needed to significantly change posterior probability. In this respect, the randomized clinical trial does not constitute a neutral algorithm for determining whether a clinical intervention is effective.

In clinical research, there are multiple candidates for sources of pre-trial beliefs. First, controlled evidence from earlier clinical trials can play a role. Second, personal clinical evidence, such as case reports, historical surveys, and anecdotal reports, can play a role. Third, accepted clinical guidelines are usually considered credible. Fourth, theoretical background knowledge and considerations regarding underlying mechanisms play important roles. Finally, basic science provides clinical researchers with evidence obtained through laboratory models. It is, however, by no means clear how the manifold sources should be weighted for the individual decision maker and which decisions should be taken when several individuals are involved. When it comes to complementary/alternative therapies, very different pre-trial beliefs can be found, for example, among clinical researchers, complementary/alternative practitioners, politicians, medical experts, patient spokesmen, and the pharmaceutical industry. We find that such differences in pre-trial beliefs at least partly can explain why there has been no consensus on how to interpret the homeopathy review referred to above.[18]

The nonneutrality of the process of interpretation challenges the claim for objectivity in clinical research. To allow subjectivity to play a role in decision making immediately calls for attempts to control contingency and explains why Bayesian reasoning is not always very popular within clinical research. On the one hand, there is no objective way to "construct" a prior probability. On the other hand, it is warranted to impose some constraints on pre-trial beliefs to protect interpretations of results from being determined by all sorts of irrelevant considerations. One interesting approach to the problem is suggested by the philosopher Wesley Salmon, who summed up his position with the notion of "tempered personalism."[19] Salmon attempted to constrain prior probabilities by plausibility arguments and stated three criteria for enhancing the prior probability of a given hypothesis:

1. *the pragmatic criteria:* the hypothesis should be advanced by serious scientists;
2. *the formal criteria:* the hypothesis should exhibit internal consistency and should be compatible with accepted laws and theories;
3. *the material criteria:* the structure of the hypothesis should be simple and be analogous to currently accepted theories.

We admit that Salmon's criteria for enhancing prior probability are too vague to act safely upon, and that much research has to be done on this subject, but we find that his approach is a promising point of departure for further considerations of the challenge from subjectivity. Moreover, we find that Salmon's criteria help clarify why many medical researchers ascribe a very low prior probability to certain complementary/alternative interventions.

What Happens If Prior Probability Is Zero?
It should be realized that in a clinical trial, the hypothesis tested is a hypothesis about a therapeutic effect and not a hypothesis about an underlying mechanism. However, when making the decision regarding how to interpret clinical trials, there is an intimate relation between the probability of the underlying mechanism and the estimated prior probability of the intervention to have important clinical effects. We agree with Vickers that prior belief should not be "the sole judge of

research," but if the postulated underlying mechanism is implausible the prior probability of the intervention to have clinical effects is reduced.[20] If the underlying mechanism is considered absurd or suffers from serious internal inconsistencies, the prior probability of the intervention to have significant clinical effects falls toward zero.

An interesting problem arises when the postulated underlying mechanism is ascribed a prior probability of zero. In such cases, the interpretation of new evidence breaks down. Conceptually, it is not meaningful to ascribe effects to absurd interventions. This point was stressed by Vandenbroucke in his *Lancet* editorial, where he stated that "Bayesian investigators will remain unimpressed by the results of homeopathy trials; when there is no convincing theory underlying a trial, the results remain uninterpretable."[21] It is important to note that exactly the same type of argumentation was used in favor of a positive interpretation by Vallance, who stated that "to assign a P(H) of 0 as an a-priori position is incompatible with rational science and Bayesian theory."[22] This statement presupposes that the postulated mechanism is ascribed a prior probability exceeding zero.

Absurd or Not Fully Explained Mechanisms

In discussing prior probabilities in complementary/alternative interventions, we find it useful to distinguish between mechanisms not fully understood and mechanisms obviously absurd.[23] If a postulated mechanism is absurd according to standard scientific position, there is a tendency to ascribe a prior probability of zero to a hypothesis about therapeutic effects, for example in the case of homeopathy. Results from trials in this situation are, as discussed above, impossible to interpret.

Other complementary/alternative therapies, for example acupuncture, are also based on theories foreign to conventional science, but are not obviously absurd: physiological responses caused by the insertion of needles on certain spots are not necessarily incompatible with standard scientific thinking. Therefore, the prior probability of acupuncture to have clinical effects exceeds zero and, thus, results from clinical trials become interpretable. In this aspect, acupuncture resembles many other complementary/alternative interventions, for example herbs and various forms of massage and manipulations. If high-quality trials repeatedly find clinically important effects of interventions with background mechanisms not understood (but not absurd either), the posterior probability will rise considerably. (See the discussion of these issues by David Hufford in this volume.)

Chance Findings: p-values and Statistical Significance

Results from a clinical trial are usually presented after a statistical analysis. The main aim of such analysis is to estimate the probability that the result of a trial was a chance finding. This is usually expressed through a p-value, which is the probability of a given result or a more extreme result, assuming the so-called null hypothesis. A null hypothesis describes a theoretical situation where the trial has no bias and the intervention no effect, and thus any positive result will be a chance event.

If a p-value is low, the probability of the result being a chance event is low. However, a problem arises: how low should a p-value be before it becomes reasonable to reject the null hypothesis and thus conclude that the result of the trial is not a chance event? There is a long-standing tradition in medical statistics that p-values under 0.05 are required to reject the null hypothesis. Results with p-values under 0.05 are often called "statistically significant findings," implying that the level of "statistical significance" has been reached. A fixed level of statistical significance is a useful practice; however, it is important to emphasize that there is no statistical or logical reason for choosing exactly 5 percent. Any specific level of statistical significance is a convention, which reflects habit and not any fundamental mathematical principle. The scientific community could just as well choose to operate with other levels of statistical significance, for example 1 percent or 10 percent. A level of statistical significance of 5 percent implies that a statistically significant result will occur just by chance in one out of twenty studies of interventions with no real effect (assuming no bias). Of course, the conventional level of statistical significance is an important factor when deciding to accept or reject a null hypothesis. However, in a situation where pre-trial beliefs about an effect are very low, there could be strong reason for assuming that a positive result was a chance finding, despite "statistical significance."

Another important aspect is that even if the interpreter decides to reject the null hypothesis because of a "statistically significant result," thus accepting that the findings of the trial were not random events, this does not automatically imply that the intervention tested has an effect. No claims about true therapeutic effects can be derived from even the most complex statistical analysis unless the risk of bias has been addressed. In this sense, the interpretation of the statistical analysis and the methodological analysis are intertwined. To conclude that an intervention has an effect is at the end of the day an "exclusion diagnosis" in that it requires both the risks of chance finding and bias to be low.

In short, the statistical analysis can provide the interpreter with the crude numbers, but that is all. Two vital decisions rest with the interpreter. One is to decide whether the finding is a random event or not; that is, to accept or reject the null hypothesis. The second is to decide whether a "statistically significant result" was biased, as discussed above.

Immunization Strategies and Further Research

We find that it is reasonable to be cautious when interpreting results from trials of complementary/alternative interventions. First, the clinical research is generally of low quality and thus has a high risk of biased results. Second, the low or moderate scientific plausibility of many of the postulated mechanisms of complementary/alternative interventions implies that prior probability in many cases is estimated to be low, and thus the posterior probability does not change dramatically despite new positive evidence.

We do not think this necessarily introduces an unfair double standard when it comes to the appraisal of randomized trials. It is reasonable to be sceptical of clinical research that generally is of low standard, regardless of whether it comes from mainstream medicine or complementary/alternative medicine. Similarly, it is always relevant to reflect on the scientific plausibility of background mechanisms in any trial. Though Bayesian reasoning clearly involves a certain degree of conservatism, this could have both positive and negative consequences. A critical cautiousness serves to protect medical practice from ineffective or even harmful treatments, whereas an exaggerated scepticism could impede the acceptance of controversial but effective treatments.

There is a tendency for both mainstream medicine and complementary/alternative medicine to embark on immunization strategies. Strong believers of complementary/alternative interventions will say that negative results from randomized trials are not important because "we just know this works." Similarly, strong sceptics will say that "if randomized trials of complementary/alternative interventions demonstrate positive effects, the randomized trials must be biased because the intervention cannot work." One way around such breakdown of communication is high-quality research. The importance of randomized trials and research into the postulated mechanisms of complementary/alternative interventions has been stressed repeatedly.[24] High-quality randomized trials with sufficient logistical back-up that are conducted by researchers who are neither strong believers nor strong sceptics would clearly be an improvement.

However, the request for more randomized trials investigating complementary/alternative interventions calls for some reflection. First, it is practically impossible to prove that an intervention has no effect at all. Therefore, there is a limit to the number of trials that it is reasonable to conduct when no clinically important effect can be found.

Second, to conduct a clinical trial implies allocation of significant intellectual and economic resources. If the pre-trial belief is very low, the enrollment of patients and allocation of resources raises both ethical and socioeconomic problems. It is not ethically defensible to include patients in studies where the likelihood of effect is very low. Such practice would violate the doctor's obligation to choose a therapy believed to be in the patient's best interest. In several countries, government-supported complementary/alternative research programs have been initiated based on strong positive beliefs among some politicians and groups of patients. Such strong beliefs among political decision makers can possibly justify allocation of resources, but it cannot solve the ethical dilemma imposed on the clinical researchers. Ideally, "equipoise" regarding preferences for the interventions being tested should be prevalent. But a tension between the "individual equipoise" of the researcher and the "community equipoise" of the scientific community (or other groups) can emerge.[25] The methodological problems can, to some extent, be redressed by balancing the research group between strong sceptics and strong believers. However, the ethical dilemma remains for the individual strong believers or sceptics in the group.

Furthermore, the allocation of significant economic resources for the investigation of treatments where no effect is expected calls for clear justifications. In the homeopathy debate, Langman questioned whether the diversion of significant resources to support trials investigating homeopathy is justified without a rational basis for choosing homeopathy.[26] However, further investigations into homeopathy have been defended by reference to the need for valid information on which to make decisions and the widespread use of homoeopathy.[27] It can be argued that allocation of resources is justified by the attempt to show certain therapies to have no effects. But, besides the difficulties in demonstrating that interventions have no effects, it is still doubtful whether strong believers among users will change their habits based on negative results.

Summary

We have discussed general issues of the interpretation of results from randomized trials of complementary/alternative interventions. In the first part of the chapter, we summarized several reviews that found the general methodological quality of complementary/alternative trials to be low, indicating a substantial risk of bias. It is therefore prudent to interpret results of randomized trials of complementary/alternative interventions cautiously, especially when trials have design inadequacies, but also when trials are conducted without appropriate logistics and when trial investigators are strong believers or strong sceptics. In the second part of the chapter we concluded that, from a Bayesian perspective, it is rational to interpret results from randomized trials conservatively when pre-trial belief in effect is low. If pre-trial belief is zero, results remain uninterpretable. If pre-trial belief exceeds zero but is still low, more positive evidence is needed. If the likelihood of a clinically important effect for an intervention is regarded as very low, the quest for more randomized trials raises ethical as well as socioeconomic problems.

NOTES

1. David M. Eisenberg et al., "Trends in Alternative Medicine Use in the United States, 1990–1997: Results of a Follow-up National Survey," *JAMA* 280, no. 18 (1998): 1569–75.

2. Stuart J. Pocock, *Clinical Trials: A Practical Approach* (Chichester, England: John Wiley & Sons, 1983).

3. Andrew Vickers et al., "How Should We Research Unconventional Therapies?" *International Journal of Technology Assessment in Health Care* 13, no. 1 (1997): 111–21.

4. Andrew Vickers, "Evidence-Based Medicine and Complementary Medicine," ACP *Journal Club* 130, no. 2 (1999): A13–A14.

5. Graham A. Colditz, James N. Miller, and Frederick Mosteller, "How Study Design Affects Outcome in Comparisons of Therapy: I: Medicine," *Statistics in Medicine* 8, no. 4 (1989): 441–54; James N. Miller, Graham A. Colditz, and Fredrick Mosteller, "How Study Design Affects Outcome in Comparisons of Therapy: II: Surgical," *Statistics in Medicine* 8, no. 4 (1989): 455–66; John D. Emerson et al., "An Empirical Study of the Possible Relation of Treatment Differences to Quality Scores in Controlled Randomized Clinical Trials," *Controlled Clinical Trials* 11, no. 5 (1990): 339–52.

6. Kenneth F. Schulz et al., "Empirical Evidence of Bias: Dimensions of Methodological Quality Associated with Estimates of Treatment Effects in Controlled Trials," *JAMA* 273, no. 5 (1995): 408–12.

7. David Moher et al., "Does Quality of Reports of Randomised Trials Affect Estimates of Intervention Efficacy Reported in Meta-analyses?" *Lancet* 352 (August 22, 1998): 609–13.

8. Bernard S. Bloom et al., "Evaluation of Randomized Controlled Trials on Complementary and Alternative Medicine," *International Journal of Technology Assessment in Health Care* 16, no. 1 (2000): 13–21.

9. Gerben ter Riet, Jos Kleinen, and Poul Knipschild, "Acupuncture and Chronic Pain: A Criteria-Based Meta-Analysis," *Journal of Clinical Epidemiology* 43, no. 11 (1990): 1191–99.

10. Klaus Linde et al., "Are the Clinical Effects of Homoeopathy Placebo Effects? A Meta-Analysis of Placebo-Controlled Trials," *Lancet* 350 (September 20, 1997): 834–43.

11. Andrew Vickers, "Clinical Trials of Homeopathy and Placebo: Analysis of a Scientific Debate," *Journal of Alternative and Complementary Medicine* 6, no. 1 (2000): 49–56.

12. Klaus Linde et al., "Impact of Study Quality on Outcome in Placebo-Controlled Trials of Homeopathy," *Journal of Clinical Epidemiology* 52, no. 7 (1999): 631–36.

13. Jürgen Margraf et al., "How 'Blind' Are Double-Blind Studies?" *Journal of Consulting and Clinical Psychology* 59, no. 1 (1991): 184–87.

14. Bert Spilker, *Guide to Clinical Trials* (New York: Raven Press, 1991), pp. 449–56.

15. International Committee of Medical Journal Editors, "Uniform Requirements for Manuscripts Submitted to Biomedical Journals," *Nordisk Medicin* 112, no. 2 (1997): 55–60.

16. Christina Turner and George J. Spilich, "Research into Smoking or Nicotine and Human Cognitive Performance: Does the Source of Funding Make a Difference?" *Addiction* 92, no. 11 (1997): 1423–26.

17. A. Caso Marasco et al., "Double-Blind Study of a Multivitamin Complex Supplemented with Ginseng Extract," *Drugs under Experimental and Clinical Research* 22, no. 6 (1996): 323–29.

18. Linde et al., "Are the Clinical Effects of Homeopathy Placebo Effects?" pp. 834–43.

19. Wesley Salmon, "Rationality and Objectivity in Science, or Tom Kuhn Meets Tom Bayes," *Minnesota Studies in the Philosophy of Science* 14 (1990): 175–204.

20. Vickers, "Clinical Trials of Homeopathy and Placebo," pp. 49–56.

21. Jan P. Vandenbroucke, "Homoeopathy Trials: Going Nowhere," *Lancet* 350 (September 20, 1997): 824.

22. Aaron K. Vallance and Kim A. Jobst, "Meta-Analysis of Homoeopathy Trials," *Lancet* 351 (January 31, 1998): 365–66.

23. Jan P. Vandenbroucke, "Medical Journals and the Shaping of Medical Knowledge," *Lancet* 352 (December 19, 1998): 2001–2006.

24. Linde et al., "Are the Clinical Effects of Homeopathy Placebo Effects?"

25. Fred Gifford, "Community-Equipoise and the Ethics of Randomized Clinical Trials," *Bioethics* 9, no. 2 (1995): 127–48.

26. M. J. Langman, "Homoeopathy Trials: Reason for Good Ones But Are They Warranted?" *Lancet* 350 (September 20, 1997): 825.

27. Linde et al., "Are the Clinical Effects of Homeopathy Placebo Effects?"; Jos Kleijnen, Paul Knipschild, and Gerben ter Riet, "Clinical Trials of Homeopathy," *British Medical Journal* 302, no. 6772 (1991): 316–23.

Wayne B. Jonas

Evidence, Ethics, and the Evaluation of Global Medicine

Western science has changed medicine radically over the last one hundred years and has come to dominate all thinking about disease and treatment in modern times. This has occurred primarily because of advances in technology and the application of the experimental method in biology and clinical testing. Our forefathers and mothers died often and early from epidemics of infectious disease, trauma, or malnutrition. Many in developing countries of the world still do. The scientific (here defined as the experimental) method, empowered with technology, has improved public health in industrialized countries tremendously. The primary advances have come in areas where a clear physical cause has been identified as being linked to a condition, such as in infectious disease (vaccines, antibiotics, and water treatments), and with the surgical management of trauma and the chemical modification of cell and body function (nutrient supplements, anesthesia, and drug treatments). As a result of these discoveries, the main concerns of our ancestors have largely diminished and we are living longer and more functional lives. The conditions that now plague most Western countries are chronic conditions reflective of these aging populations.

Medical Science and Globalization

Modern medicine is largely an invention of Western cultures. While it succeeds dramatically in many areas, such as the control of acute and infectious disease, it also fails in others, such as the management of chronic conditions with complex etiologies. It has mastered the cure, but struggles with the care—and it costs too much. Its successes and failures have arisen largely from a focus on science as defined by laboratory and experimental methods and it is empowered by technology. A singular orientation of research methods toward the experimental method for defining what is valuable in medicine accompanies this success. However, forces such as information technology, the increasing democratization of medicine, migration of peoples, the speed of travel, and the subsequent globalization of cultural concepts once isolated to certain parts of the world have opened a new challenge for this approach to medicine. Basic assumptions about the building blocks of the world and the nature of life, health, disease, and treatment are now opening up to the diversity of concepts in the world's healing traditions.

When these healing traditions come into the West they are placed in the category of complementary and alternative medicine (CAM) and considered "unscientific." Some of these systems of medicine are thousands of years old, and they embody societal and individual perceptions. Can the singular orientation of research methods in the West still be justified in such a world? Is it causing harm by limiting the development of new medical approaches and scientific strategies? Does the imposition of a singular orientation—one that is controlled primarily by those who do research—have ethical implications for the principles of equity and respect for persons? Can it and should it be sustained in an increasingly globalized world? If not, is it possible to develop a pluralistic approach to research methods that retains the value of Western science for medicine and yet respects the diversity of radically different concepts about life, health, and disease?

In his chapter in this book, "Assessments of Efficacy in Biomedicine: The Turn toward Methodological Pluralism," Kenneth Schaffner summarizes the situation: "So, not only do there appear to be different kinds of studies that might be done, and diverse ends to which different studies may be put, but for some the whole framework of experimental study design . . . and its underlying ontologies and methodologies may be foreign to the CAM approach."

A Model for Scientific Pluralism

In this chapter I outline a model for research strategies that attempts to be true to the core scientific advances of the past century and yet allows for a more balanced role for research methods often considered secondary to experimental approaches. The model balances experimental and observational designs and outlines three levels of investigation within each of those designs preferred by public audiences, resulting in six approaches. It suggests that the definition of "scientifically established" should involve the provision of information using all six of these approaches. I illustrate first how assumptions about causality from a global perspective in medicine require that both experimental and observational approaches be used in the evaluation of medical "facts." Using an unbalanced strategy creates dilemmas in the treatment of chronic disease that cannot be addressed by simply "better" or "more rigorous" experimental studies. I discuss the ethical reasons for having a "balanced" instead of a "better" scientific strategy and suggest that the former orientation is more useful for defining the role of science in global medicine.

Cause and the Hierarchy of Evidence

The fundamental assumption inherent in the experimental method is that determination of direct cause and effect links between variables is the primary and sufficient goal of most biomedical research. This assumption has proved so powerful for addressing the diseases of the past century that it has become dogmatically and universally applied to all areas of medicine and much of psychology. Experimental methods initially used in the laboratory were gradually adopted for testing new therapies, using experiments on humans. In clinical research this led to the development and adoption of the randomized controlled trial (RCT) as the "gold standard" against which all other methods are now compared.[1] Evaluation criteria have been developed using this standard and are often called "internal validity" criteria. These include the creation of hypotheses based on studies of postulated "mechanisms" of linear causality, selection of subjects to ensure homogeneous diagnostic and measurement categories, blind and random allocation of subjects to comparison groups, objective and complete outcome measurement, proper statistical and power calculations to minimize chance findings, and often blinding of all participants in order to control for expectation bias.[2]

The dominance of biomedicine's search for causal links between variables has led to the current "hierarchy of evidence." Figure 1 depicts this typical hierarchy, in which the RCT (or the systematic review of RCTs) is above all other research approaches; cohort studies, observational and epidemiological studies, and case series and reports are subservient to this design and its goal. Thus, we refer to the value of observational data as "hypothesis generating" and descriptive information as useful for "deciding when an RCT should be done." Justification for the use of observational data is also oriented around how well one can make it approximate an experiment.[3]

Fancy statistical methods have been developed to help "control" for possible causal confounders in observational trials, and consistency

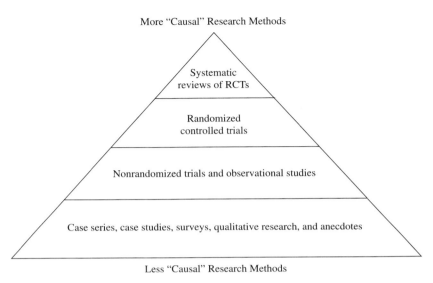

Figure 1. The Hierarchy of Evidence

between findings in observational and experimental trials is used to justify the validity of the observational data. When disparities are found between observational and experimental research, the observational data is usually considered wrong.[4]

Practice and the Hierarchy of Evidence

The assumption that we must find specific causal links between treatments and outcomes flows over into medical practice, defining what we agree "works" and what does not. Physicians are taught that clinical research using the experimental design at the top of this evidence pyramid (the systematic review of RCTs and individual RCTs) is the "best evidence" for accepting a therapy and should be sought out in making clinical decisions. In "evidence-based medicine," the goal is to use the information derived from the top of this hierarchy.[5] Any clinical information from the lower levels of this pyramid (case-controlled trial or observational research and case series) is considered suspect and may even be dismissed. Electronic search strategies for improving the efficiency of evidence-based medicine in clinical practice seek to filter out all but RCTs and systematic reviews (SRs) or meta-analyses of RCTs for consideration when evaluating the evidence for what "works."[6]

Reimbursement and health policy practices also frequently use this strategy.

This strategy works well in many clinical situations, especially when strong causal links turn out to exist between treatment and outcomes, when the measurement occurs within the testing timeframe, and when the effects of treatment are largely additive so that simple statistical comparisons can be made. The application of an RCT design is most likely to be useful when tight cause and effect links exist between variables. Table 1 lists the conditions under which RCTs are most likely to achieve their goal of attribution and thus when internal validity criteria are most attainable. This occurs under the assumption that precise testing for specific causality is the most important goal for research. The conditions for an RCT are most often met when a disease occurs over a short period of time and involves single domains so that multiple confounding factors have little time to influence the outcome.

This type of research design best fits the assumptions of the biomedical model inherent in drug testing, where tight cause and effect links can be measured under blind conditions. It works well in acute disease with short duration, with single treatments that are easily standardized, and when the effects are additive—as when a chemical treatment is

Table 1. Preconditions for Successful RCTs

Diagnosis	well-defined
	discrete
Intervention	lack of evidence
	simple
	relatively short
	content-based (as opposed to process-based)
	additive
Outcome	agreed on by all participants
	easily defined and measured
Specificity of intervention	essential to establish
	basis for large-scale, population-based, and public health decisions
Alternatives	lacking
	fraught with risk or side-effects
	ineffective
Preferences	none on part of doctors, patients, or investigators

compared to nothing. This approach is sometimes referred to as the "regulatory" model of intervention testing because it has been applied most intensively for the regulation of drug marketing. However, internal validity criteria are not so useful and may even hinder the collection of useful information in diverse public health settings. That is, these studies may not have much external validity, or value outside the study situation.[7]

Balancing the Hierarchy of Evidence

Those involved in health services research and technology assessment often recognize that observational research can produce data that have value on their own. Non-RCT designs, by contrast, are usually described in terms of their ability to supplement or guide RCT investigation and data. An exception to this is in the attempt to more clearly distinguish between "efficacy" and "effectiveness" research as outlined by the Agency for Healthcare Research and Quality. Efficacy refers to evidence that a therapy produced an effect in an experimental setting (thus demonstrating a cause and effect link of a treatment to an outcome), and effectiveness refers to an assessment of the impact of an intervention in normal clinical practice (where causal links cannot be identified). Making this distinction reminds us that the value of causation found in RCTs needs to be checked for its usefulness with observational and health services research. Recently, the National Institute of Mental Health of the National Institutes of Health (NIH) has called for more expanded research methods to bridge the gap between efficacy sought in experimental research and data from observational studies to inform treatment practice in a community.[8]

A more explicit "balance" in research and evaluation strategies between the criteria of internal validity (focused on identifying causal links) and external validity (focused on clarifying impact and utility) is needed.[9] This would shift the single orientation to a dual orientation in research methods. Rather than assuming that studies with high internal validity are "better" than others (the hierarchy approach), a dual orientation recognizes that both internal and external validity have intrinsic value and different purposes. Understanding assumptions about causality in both Western medicine and non-Western systems of medicine is important for expanding this dual orientation and seeking "methodological balance" in a global medicine perspective.

"Holistic" and Acausality Concepts
in Global Medicine Research

Chronic Disease and the Systems Model in Medicine

Many chronic diseases, complex treatment systems, and nonadditive interactions between them do not follow the assumptions of tight cause-effect links. Most chronic conditions are produced by multiple interacting influences (webs of "causation"), and many interventions do not produce additive effects. Under these circumstances the experimental method becomes insensitive and misleading and requires a more "holistic" and nonreductionistic approach to evaluation. The importance of addressing complexity, nonlinearity, and holistic aspects in biology and medicine is being explored in a number of areas including epidemiology,[10] molecular biology,[11] physiology,[12] clinical medicine,[13] and clinical trials.[14] The "biopsychosocial" model of medicine described by Engel thirty years ago is an attempt to frame how this complexity is handled clinically.[15] The dialectic between a reductionistic and holistic orientation in research strategies in biology has been an important subtext in biomedicine for the past one hundred years.[16]

Confusion Produced by Causality Dominance

A number of authors have discussed how a strictly causal orientation to disease and illness also creates difficulties in the design and interpretation of clinical trials.[17] There are many examples of the confusion and ambiguity that arise from making the identification of specific causal links the primary goal of clinical research. These include: (1) the difficulty in determining if antidepressants "work,"[18] (2) the variable effects of established drug treatments for ulcer disease showing that they "work" in one country but do not in another,[19] (3) the inability of the RCT method to determine whether homeopathy has any specific activity or not,[20] (4) the failure of many "proven" (by RCTs) and effective drug treatments to provide long-term benefit in common chronic conditions such as arthritis, cancer, and heart disease,[21] (5) the severely restricted scope of what can be "proved" to be better than placebo in complex interventions such as behavioral medicine, acupuncture, physiotherapy, surgery, etc., (6) the confusion produced by RCT research of many nondrug therapies where the "active" treatment cannot be shown to be superior to the control conditions yet is clearly superior to no treatment or to simpler, proven therapies,[22] and (7) the continued dominance of expensive and highly invasive surgical therapies for chronic disease when the dramatic impact they produce cannot be and is not tested for its causal specificity.[23] Thus, different scientific criteria are applied to different types of treatments and the value of evidence is undermined.

The Clinical Consequences of Causality Dominance

Most primary care physicians involved in longitudinal care see both the value and limitations of using a causal model for the care of patients on a continual basis. The model works well for conditions of bacterial infection, trauma, surgically correctable lesions, and for manipulation of physiology, such as reduction of blood pressure and acute pain. It does not work well for many chronic conditions and functional problems. Any physician attempting to practice "evidence-based medicine" sees the failure of the experimental orientation in providing useful answers to these more complex situations. In the appendix I have used a typical case of medical management over a lifecycle to illustrate how this approach often "works" and "does not work" over time, depending entirely on one's evidence preference.

Correspondences and Acausality in CAM Systems

There is an additional assumption about causality that is inherent in many CAM and traditional medical systems that goes beyond the systems model perspective just discussed. Most major traditional medical systems outside the West do not share the assumption that causal links or probability assessment are always the most important goal of investigation or that they provide the most useful approach for treatment of disease. Some systems, such as traditional Chinese medicine (TCM), are based not on assumptions of linear causation but on the concept of "correspondences."[24] The correspondences model assumes that events occurring at one level of a system (psychological and biological, for example) are simultaneously linked to changes at other levels (social or environmental). The correspondences concept does not deny that linear causality exists but assumes that causal links can vary and be influenced on any level of the system. Thus, chronic headaches may be due to vasoconstriction, but they may be altered by rearrangement of the diet or furniture in the house, even if one cannot demonstrate statistically that such alteration occurs in the aggregate or will occur at another time when conditions are different. "Correspondences" between systems can alter not only outcomes but the strength of the established causal links. If the strength of causal links can be altered by contextual influences, then the value of finding such primary causal links diminishes.

Other traditional systems have similar but even more radical assumptions about causality. Ayurvedic medicine assumes that "universal consciousness" can fundamentally alter medical conditions and so is the appropriate focus of therapy. Aspects of consciousness are not simply causal but "creative" and can alter the tightness of causal links and the outcomes of disease, as well as creating new links and associations that did not previously exist.[25] In other words, they are acausal in the sense that they decouple causal links and create new ones. Recent experimental data on distant healing and experiments on nonlocality indicate that, under certain circumstances, a "creative" process that interacts with causality may occur.[26]

Under conditions of acausality it is not possible for the experimental method always to be useful. Causal treatment–outcome links found under some experiments may disappear in other experiments, yet other links can emerge from the conscious (or in some systems the "spiritual") interaction of participants and environment and time. Native American medicine also assumes the relativity of causal links and takes a "spiritual" interpretation of this interaction, in which the environment (animals, rocks, plants, etc.) plays an integral part in the decoupling of causality.[27] Acausal models have been proposed for other, more recent systems of unconventional medicine such as Rogers's theory of nursing[28] and homeopathy.[29] If we are to incorporate these assumptions into a global medicine research, clearly an expanded approach to research is needed in which causality, probability, and acausality are nonexclusive dimensions of our evaluation strategy.

Models of Causality, Complexity, and Acausality in Practice and Research

Figure 2 illustrates how causality, probability (systems theory), and acausality can be visualized in practice. On the left side of the figure are listed a variety of disease "agents" and influences arranged in a systems hierarchy from social to molecular. The "host" (an individual, population, or ecosystem) with which these agents interact is represented by the oval in the middle of the figure. The "responses" (a symptom, illness, disease rate, or outcome measure) of the interaction are listed on the right side of the figure.

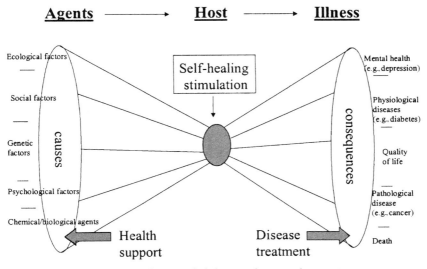

Figure 2. Causality, Probability, and Acausality in Practice

Take a clinical example: If an "agent" has a tight link to an invariant response by the "host," then a causal approach works well both for researching this link and for using this causal understanding in treatment. The dark line illustrates this situation. A blow to the head causing a skull fracture is an example of a very tight causal link. Exposure to streptoccocus bacteria causing a sore throat and smoking causing lung disease are examples of moderately tight links. The contribution of blood pressure, cholesterol levels, and depression to cardiovascular disease are examples of looser and more variable links. Social and behavioral factors usually influence a multitude of risk factors and diseases. They cannot be captured by connecting single links to single diseases but influence almost every link (and disease) in our model.

Causal models look for specific treatments (the magic bullet), probabilistic models (systems) look for wide and general medical effects (general medical effectiveness), and acausal models look for methods of altering these associations—often by creating new meanings (causal links) that are not dependent on classical time and space relationships. The application of causal principles to "tight link" situations works well. The application of causal principles to "weak link" situations does not and may result in adverse effects and undesired consequences. Under these conditions, the application of a causal model is not only ineffective, it produces undesired adverse effects and high costs. In these circumstances a systems or acausal model may be more appropriate (see Appendix, p. 144).

Evaluation Ethics in Global Medicine

While global medicine will require a broadening of our concepts of causation, it will also require a more comprehensive approach to the ethics of research methods and the medical information those methods provide. By this I do not mean improved informed consent, privacy safeguards, or better ensurance of equipoise in clinical trials, all of which are important. By the ethics of methodological balance I mean that global medicine research will need to pay closer attention to the values that various audiences place on information. Traditionally, medical ethics requires that beneficence, nonmaleficence, autonomy, justice, and a respect for persons be an integral part of all medical care. Evaluation ethics requires that our research and evaluation tools also serve these purposes. If we respect the value preferences that various audiences have for different types of information, then we should "balance" our research strategies with the methods necessary to provide that information. The conventional hierarchy of evidence depicted in Figure 1 is a research strategy oriented toward the select group of basic and clinical scientists who conduct research. To "balance" this strategy is to use research approaches that also respect the information preferences of other audiences. This means that we commit to using research methods that provide the information audiences other than scientists and clinical researchers value and seek.

The Audience and the Evidence

While all groups ultimately are interested in all types of information, most groups see certain types of information as primary and seek it out.[30] The following are some of the main audiences that research serves and the type of information they often see as primary.

- *Patients* who are ill, or their family members, often want to hear details about other individuals with similar illnesses who have used a treatment and recovered. If the treatment appears to be safe and there is little risk of harm from it, evidence from these stories may convince them to use the treatment. This type of evidence is called anecdotal, or case reports.

- *Practitioners,* who see many patients, realize that what works in one case may not work in another, and they need more than a few patient recovery stories to recommend a therapy. They often want to know what the likelihood or probability is that a patient will recover or have an adverse effect based on a series of similar patients who have received the treatment in actual practice. For example, out of one hundred patients with a condition who received a treatment, did 20 percent or 80 percent improve and how many had side effects? They also want to know about any difficulties in using the therapy, including its cost and inconvenience. This type of evidence comes from observational or clinical outcomes data.

- *Clinical researchers* usually want to know how much improvement occurred in a group who received the treatment compared to another group who did not receive the treatment. If 80 percent of patients who received a treatment got better, did 75 percent of similar patients get better just from coming to the doctor and getting any treatment? If so, only 5 percent of the improvement would be attributed to the treatment. This is comparative clinical trial evidence. Some scientists will only accept comparative evidence for a treatment if it has come from an experiment in which blinding and randomization have been followed. This is clinical experimental or randomized controlled trial evidence.

- *Basic scientists* may want objective evidence supporting a mechanism of action from laboratory experiments that can explain the effects observed in clinical research or guide better clinical research. This is basic science evidence.

- *Policymakers,* or those in charge of determining public laws and policy, often need definitive "proof" that a practice is safe and effective. They require evidence on which a high degree of confidence can be placed since errors made in policy can adversely affect millions of people and cost billions of dollars. This type of evidence comes from extensive evaluation and synthesis of several research reports through systematic reviews, meta-analyses, and consensus evaluations from experts in the field.

Each of these evidence preferences is legitimate for the purposes and audiences it serves. An ethical approach to development of research strategies would acknowledge the legitimacy of those preferences and seek to produce each of these types of information. If we make one type of evidence the "gold standard" and orient our research approaches toward that approach, we not only assume that type of information is the only valid goal for research to pursue, we preferentially serve only a few audiences and their goals to the neglect of others.

An Evidence House for Global Medicine

How are we to construct a research and evaluation strategy for global medicine that encompasses the causal, systems, and acausal assumptions of various world views and also provides information valued by diverse audiences? The ethical application of science to systems so varied in global medicine will require an evaluation approach that encompasses evidence in a number of domains. Instead of orienting our research methods in a fashion subservient to assumptions of causation only, I suggest that our methods be arrayed in a structure wherein each method is more clearly linked to the type of information it provides (Figure 3). Such a structure distinguishes between research methods that seek to isolate causal links (effects testing on the left of Figure 3), and those methods that look for clinical impact where complex or acausal assumptions apply (utility testing on the right of Figure 3). This structure also respects the information preferences sought by various audiences and acknowledges their intrinsic contribution to medical knowledge. It also allows for scientific evidence and its ethical application to remain as the foundation of medicine. Yet it provides the flexibility to ask an expanded set of questions in the context of the differing assumptions about causation and the diverse values placed on information.

Research Methods for a Balanced Evidence House

Figure 3 illustrates six methods of research that are used in the investigation of medicine and the type of information that these approaches generally provide. Note that these research types have a semi-hierarchical structure in which the foundational methods at the bottom address theory and meaning, respectively, which are built upon by the methods above them through progressively complex levels of observation and experimentation. While there are many variations on these methods,

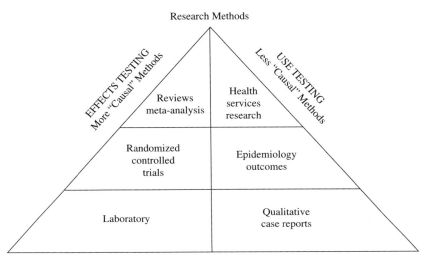

Figure 3. Balanced Evidence Hierarchy

I feel that these form a core set that can serve as a foundation for a global medicine research strategy.

The core methods include:

1. *Qualitative research,* such as detailed case studies and patient interviews, that describe diagnostic and treatment approaches and investigate patient preferences and relevance of those approaches. Qualitative approaches have been extensively developed in the nursing profession and social sciences and are becoming increasingly common in primary care.

2. *Laboratory and basic science approaches* that investigate the basic mechanisms and biological plausibility of practices; *in vitro* (cell culture and molecular models) and *in vivo* (testing in normal, disease prone, or genetically altered animals), and mixed approaches are now used extensively.

3. *Observational studies,* such as practice audit, outcomes research, and other types of observational research, that describe associations between interventions and outcomes. Practice audit involves monitoring outcomes on all or a selected sample of patients that receive treatment, with evaluation before and after an intervention to measure effects. These studies may not have a comparison group, or comparison groups may be developed

by sampling patients not treated with the intervention from other practices or in the same practice prior to the intervention.

4. *Randomized controlled trials* attempt to isolate or compare the specific contribution of different interventions on outcomes. These studies usually involve the assignment of patients to one treatment group or another using a method that ensures the groups are comparable on all factors that might influence outcomes except for the treatment. Various methods are used, such as randomly selected numbers or computer-generated assignment. Treatments, without knowledge of this assignment, may or may not be evaluated and are best done by concealing knowledge of which patients will get which treatment at least at the time of assignment.

5. Methods for assessing the accuracy of these methods such as *meta-analyses, systematic reviews,* and *expert review and evaluation.* Methods for expert review and summary of research have evolved over the past several years, with systematic-protocol-driven approaches such as meta-analysis being used more frequently to increase the confidence that the effects found in clinical research are accurate and applicable across populations.

6. *Health services research* for examining the actual utility and impact of interventions in light of social factors such as access, feasibility, costs, practitioner competence, patient compliance, and so forth. Often this type of research involves surveys or sampling from groups already receiving an intervention to look at the quality and costs of the intervention, as well as other factors. Random sampling may or may not be used.

Each of these methods has its own goals and quality criteria, and each one provides a certain type of information (Figure 4). These are listed below.

1. *Mechanism and basic biological effects on and in living systems.* This is investigated through basic science and laboratory techniques and asks the question, "what happens and why?" Basic research can provide us with explanations for biological processes that are required to refine and advance our knowledge in any therapeutic field.

2. *Meaning and the examination of the subjective.* This information comes through stories, anecdotes, and descriptions of case reports. Quality research in this area, however, requires detailed

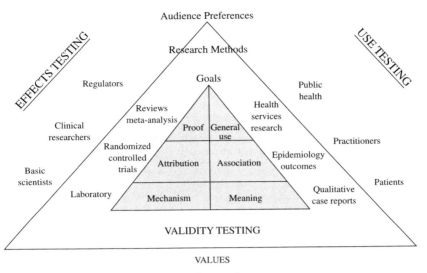

Figure 4. The Evidence House

qualitative evaluation methods, which were outlined in the qualitative evaluation section of the NIH Office of Alternative Medicine (OAM) Methodology Conference. This knowledge domain provides information about whether our efforts are taking the correct focus by incorporating patient-centered outcomes and patient preferences, which then reduces the risk of outcomes substitution (measuring irrelevant outcomes) when a therapy is applied.

3. *Attribution.* In clinical research, this is termed "efficacy" and is best obtained through research methods such as the randomized controlled trial. This domain looks for cause and effect evidence of proof and is useful when information is needed to make claims about how parts of a therapeutic system affect preselected outcomes of a clinical condition.

4. *Associations.* When the identification of cause and effect links is impractical, unethical, unreasonable, or impossible, the fourth domain of information—looking for associations—is needed. In clinical medicine this is known as "effectiveness" and involves such research methods as epidemiological and outcomes research strategies. It is best applied when one is evaluating complex, long-term, or chronic conditions. Complex systems evaluation

is needed for traditional medicine and the utility of specific therapies when applied in various clinical situations. This type of knowledge is useful when indications are the desired outcome and when one is seeking knowledge about possible adverse effects that are rare or have not been previously expected.

5. *Confidence.* This knowledge domain is explored through peer-review, systematic review, and meta-analysis of scientific literature. Its purpose is to refine and determine whether definitive proof for a phenomenon exists. It is part of, but not the whole, validation process and requires the intimate involvement of a wide peer-review process. This area, like all others, requires an objective, systematic, explicit, and comprehensive approach for valid conclusions.

6. *Generalizability.* This area involves an even wider public review process. It is desirable when the goal of that information is the acceptance and adoption of particular practices. This area deals with the evaluation of external validity aspects such as access, feasibility, use, and so forth. It primarily involves public use. Health services research provides information in this knowledge domain.

From the clinical perspective, the ultimate goal of all of these domains of knowledge is the identification of optimal medical management and the selection of what types of diagnostic or therapeutic strategies warrant direct comparative trials. From the basic biomedical perspective, the ultimate goal of all these domains is the understanding and control of the fundamental processes of life. Progress of an intervention from investigation to evaluation to validation requires a research strategy that provides a balanced portfolio feeding all of these knowledge domains. Excessive emphasis on one domain to the neglect of another will likely impede progress toward validation, violate the moral principles of justice and respect for persons, and may result in harm when applied to chronic disease and complex treatment systems.

Toward a Global Research Strategy

How does this all fit together when choosing clinical research strategies in CAM? The "Balanced Evidence Hierarchy" framework (Figure 3) can help identify the main types of research needed. The decision to pursue a particular approach then depends on a number of factors, including:

- the simplicity or complexity of the condition and therapy being investigated,
- the type of information sought (causal, descriptive, associative, etc.),
- the purpose for which a particular audience will use the information, and
- the methods of investigation that are available, ethical, and affordable.

Figure 4 illustrates how these factors align in the "Evidence House." The main purpose and audience for which a research project is undertaken can be used as the anchoring factor in determining the appropriate method. For example, in complex practices that are not well described, observational data and outcomes research or pilot trials may be the best initial approach. In well-described practices, outcomes data coupled with decision analysis may provide the best strategic approach. Natural products, whose active constituents are unknown, require consultation with expert practitioners and then laboratory characterization before controlled clinical research is done. Natural products that are well characterized may need randomized controlled trials to determine whether their potential public health impact warrants public use. Placebo studies of natural products may be more useful for making regulatory decisions (e.g., product marketing and claims) than for individual or public health decisions. The NIH's study of the efficacy of the herb St. John's wort for depression using a large, three-armed, multicentered, placebo-controlled trial is an example of this latter approach.

Outcomes research in actual practice needs more development and emphasis in certain areas. For example, a physician considering a patient referral for acupuncture might want to know what kind of patients local acupuncturists see, how they are treated, whether these patients are satisfied with treatment, and what the outcomes are. This comes from practice audit (observational research), surveys, and qualitative research.[31] Such information may be more valuable than relying on the results of small (or large) placebo-controlled trials done in another country with practitioners and populations quite different than those in the patient and physician's community. Unfortunately, methods for conducting observational studies on complex practices have been neglected in the effort to conduct randomized trials for a few, more easily tested and popular CAM products. Data collection, monitoring, and interpretation of observational studies must be at least as carefully performed as in experimental studies and so efficient systems are needed in order to ensure quality execution of such studies.

Finally, for the exploration of theories and data that do not fit into our current assumptions about causality (e.g., psychic healing and homeopathy), a carefully thought out, basic science strategy for approaching these topics is needed. Given the public interest and the implications for science of some of these areas, it is irresponsible for the scientific community to completely ignore them.[32] Using the evidence house presented here provides a place and justification for these types of research.

CAM and the Evolution of the Scientific Method

The interaction of conventional and unconventional medicine has often produced improvements in the scientific method. Fifty years ago, for example, current methods of blinding and randomization became accepted parts of orthodox medical research after they were first developed and applied to unorthodox practices such as mesmerism, psychic healing, and homeopathy in an attempt to disprove them.[33] It is doubtful that many conventional or complementary therapies will ever be fully "scientifically established"; that is, will fill in all six evidence domains of Figure 3. Decisions about what is "sufficient" evidence for particular purposes and audiences (individual, practice, regulatory, public health, etc.) will require a more careful examination of the role science plays in the management of chronic disease and in the need to investigate alternative causal "paradigms." Science answers incremental and isolated questions, and the public must understand that research can never answer all questions of interest. Since skepticism about unorthodox practices is higher than for conventional practices, a demand for more rigorous evidence than usual is often made before such practices are accepted.

At the same time, the march toward global medicine challenges us to make explicit the definition of quality and of the term "scientifically established" in medicine and to demonstrate the evidence upon which those quality criteria are based.[34] Research in CAM may help us develop the decision rules for improving research rigor and for developing a better strategic approach for medical research. Thus, the continuing interface between orthodox and unorthodox medicine today provides the opportunity for new research strategies—a balanced pluralism— to arise. By purposefully maintaining a creative (not destructive) tension between the established and the frontier we can both advance scientific methods and more clearly define the limits and purpose of the scientific process for medicine as a whole.

NOTES

1. A. Jadad, *Randomized Controlled Trials: A User's Guide* (London: BMJ Books, 1998).

2. D. Moher, "CONSORT: An Evolving Tool to Help Improve the Quality of Reports of Randomized Controlled Trials," *JAMA* 279 (1998): 1489–91.

3. D. F. Stroup et al., "Meta-analysis of Observational Studies in Epidemiology," *JAMA* 283 (2000): 2008–12.

4. M. Egger and G. D. Smith, "Misleading Meta-analysis," *British Medical Journal* 311, no. 7007 (1995): 753–54.

5. D. L. Sackett et al., *Clinical Epidemiology: A Basic Science for Clinical Medicine* (Boston: Little, Brown, 1991).

6. W. Rosenberg and A. Donald, "Evidence Based Medicine: An Approach to Clinical Problem-Solving," *British Medical Journal* 310 (1995): 1122–26 (see comments).

7. I. Kirsch and M. J. Rosandino, "Do Double-Blind Studies with Informed Consent Yield Externally Valid Results? An Empirical Test," *Psychopharmacology* 110 (1993): 437–42.

8. G. Norquist, B. Lebowitz, and S. Hyman, "Expanding the Frontier of Treatment Research," *Prevention and Treatment* 2 (1999): 0001a.

9. D. J. Miklowitz and J. F. Clarkin, "Balancing Internal and External Validity," *Prevention and Treatment* 2 (1999): 0004c.

10. M. Susser and E. Susser, "Choosing a Future for Epidemiology: II: From Black Box to Chinese Boxes and Eco-Epidemiology," *American Journal of Public Health* 86 (1996): 674–77.

11. R. C. Strohman, "Ancient Genomes, Wise Bodies, Unhealthy People: Limits of a Genetic Paradigm in Biology and Medicine," *Perspectives in Biology and Medicine* 37 (1993): 112–45; R. Strohman, "Epigenesis: The Missing Beat in Biotechnology," *Biotechnology* 12 (1994): 156–64.

12. T. Elbert et al., "Chaos and Physiology: Deterministic Chaos in Excitable Cell Assemblies," *Physiology Review* 74 (1994):1–47; L. A. Lipsitz and A. L. Goldberger, "Loss of 'Complexity' and Aging: Potential Applications of Fractal and Chaos Theory to Senescence," *JAMA* 267 (1992): 1806–09.

13. J. E. Skinner et al., "Application of Chaos Theory to Biology and Medicine," *Integrative Physiological and Behavioral Science* 27 (1992): 39–53; W. L. Miller et al., "Understanding Change in Primary Care Practice Using Complexity Theory," *Journal of Family Practice* 46 (1998): 369–76.

14. R. I. Horwitz, "Complexity and Contradiction in Clinical Trial Research," *American Journal of Medicine* 82 (1987): 498–510.

15. G. L. Engel, "The Need for a New Medical Model: A Challenge for Biomedicine," *Science* 196 (1977): 129–36.

16. C. Lawrence and G. Weisz, *Greater than the Parts: Holism in Biomedicine, 1920–1950* (Oxford: Oxford University Press, 1998).

17. Horwitz, "Complexity and Contradiction in Clinical Trial Research"; J. Heron, "Critique of Conventional Research Methodology," *Comparative Medicine Research* 1 (1986): 10–22; J. Leibrich, "Measurement of Efficacy: A Case for Holistic Research," *Comparative Medicine Research* 4 (1990): 21–25.

18. I. Kirsch and G. Spirstein, "Listening to Prozac but Hearing Placebo: A Meta-Analysis of Antidepressant Medication," *Prevention and Treatment* 1 (1998): 0002a.

19. D. E. Moerman, "Cultural Variations in the Placebo Effect: Ulcers, Anxiety, and Blood Pressure," *Medical Anthropology Quarterly* 14 (2000): 51–72.

20. K. Linde et al., "Are the Clinical Effects of Homeopathy All Placebo Effects? A Meta-analysis of Randomized, Placebo Controlled Trials," *Lancet* 350 (1997): 834–43.

21. T. Pincus, "Analyzing Long-term Outcomes of Clinical Care without Randomized Controlled Clinical Trials: The Consecutive Patient Questionnaire Database," *Advances* 13 (1997): 3–31; J. Bailar, "Cancer Undefeated," *NEJM* 336 (1997): 1569–74.

22. Anonymous, *Clinical Evidence* (London: BMJ, 2000).

23. A. G. Johnson, "Surgery as Placebo," *Lancet* 344 (1994): 1140–42.

24. M. Porkert, *The Theoretical Foundations of Chinese Medicine: Systems of Correspondence* (Cambridge: MIT Press, 1974), p. 368; L. Lao, "Traditional Chinese Medicine," in *Essentials of Complementary and Alternative Medicine,* ed. W. B. Jonas and J. S. Levin (Philadelphia: Lipincott, Williams & Wilkins, 1999), pp. 216–32.

25. V. D. Lad, "Ayurvedic Medicine," in *Essentials of Complementary and Alternative Medicine,* pp. 200–215.

26. D. I. Radin, *The Conscious Universe: The Scientific Truth behind Psychic Phenomena* (San Francisco: HarperEdge, 1997).

27. K. B. H. Cohen, "Native American Medicine," in *Essentials of Complementary and Alternative Medicine,* pp. 233–51.

28. M. E. Rogers, *An Introduction to the Theoretical Basis of Nursing* (Philadelphia: F. A. Davis, 1970).

29. H. Walach, "The Magic of Signs: A Non-local Interpretation of Homeopathy," *British Homeopathic Journal* 89, no. 3 (2000): 127–40.

30. M. Kelner and B. Wellman, *The Social Science of Complementary and Alternative Medicine* (New York: Gordon & Breach, 2001).

31. C. M. Cassidy, "Chinese Medicine Users in the United States Part I: Utilization, Satisfaction, Medical Plurality," *Journal of Alternative and Complementary Medicine* 4 (1998): 17–27; C. M. Cassidy, "Chinese Medicine Users in the United States Part II: Preferred Aspects of Care," *Journal of Alternative and Complementary Medicine* 4 (1998): 189–202.

32. W. B. Jonas, "Researching Alternative Medicine," *Nature Medicine* 3 (1997): 824–27.

33. T. J. Kaptchuk, "Intentional Ignorance: The History of Blind Assessment and Placebo Controls in Medicine," *Bulletin of the History of Medicine* 72 (1998): 389–433.

34. Stroup et al., "Meta-analysis of Observational Studies in Epidemiology."

A Clinical Example of Causality Applied Longitudinally to Chronic Conditions

The following example demonstrates what happens to a typical patient with chronic disease in which there are multiple interacting "agents" and "responses" when he is treated on the basis of the assumptions of a linear causal model developed for acute disease.

A young patient is discovered at a health screening fair to have elevated cholesterol and a high-fat, high-salt diet. The patient is sent to a medical clinic for confirmation of the cholesterol and then a dietitian gives a group or individual lecture on a low-fat diet. Usually, no individual dietary analysis is available to provide the patient with specific information about his diet composition and what needs to be altered. The relationship between other aspects of his diet (fiber and protein) and physical performance are not discussed. An exercise program is not prescribed and stress issues are not addressed to any significant degree.

The patient has significant family stress. However, because family involvement is not included in the intervention, he is unable to alter his diet significantly enough to change his cholesterol until these issues are addressed. This is especially important since it is his wife who does all of the shopping and cooking. This person's primary obstacle to dietary change may be stress and negative coping skills that cannot be effectively addressed by the dietitian. In the present system, if this patient returns to the clinic for follow-up, he is placed on cholesterol-lowering medications. The cholesterol will come down (his overall risk of dying will not), but later the family dysfunction and poor coping skills that are not addressed may result in alcohol use and elevated blood pressure. Average cost for cholesterol-lowering medications can be $1,500 per year for this patient or $75,000 for life, assuming that he lives fifty more years.

At middle age, the patient's hypertension is identified through a periodic physical, dental exam, or health risk appraisal assessment (HRAA), confirmed, and treated successfully with medications. He may be given similar cursory instructions about lifestyle as with his cholesterol intervention but without significant time or details to make effective changes. Effective, long-term interventions to assist him in stress reduction (relaxation and meditation), dietary change, exercise, and physiological control (biofeedback) are not initiated. Medical treatment of blood pressure would have an average cost for his anti-hypertensive medications of $700 per year or $28,000 for life, assuming that he lives forty more years.

Results of this patient's periodic physical checkups now look fine. The patient continues to be at increased risk for multiple problems, however, and will function at suboptimal levels of health because the underlying etiology and background causes of his currently identified problems have not been altered. The continued stress and poor coping methods and continued use of alcohol and nicotine may eventually lead to functional illness, family conflict, and increased chances of developing heart and liver disease. His job performance will likely be suboptimal. His family's medical utilization will likely be high.

If this patient were to have sudden increased stressors placed on him it is likely that he would be unable to cope both physically (because of smoking and diet effects on endurance) and psychologically (because his usual coping methods of alcohol use further impair his judgment and because family dysfunction at home increases his risk of family or self abuse). Reducing single risk factors through medication without addressing the behavioral factors that underlie those risks often results in the reduction of personal resources when this patient is challenged by increased stress.

Continued unhealthy dietary and addictive practices (now masked during his HRAA screen by cholesterol- and blood-pressure-lowering medications) such as the intake of alcohol, tobacco, and high-fat, high-salt, low-fiber, and low-nutrient foods will leave this patient at increased risk of developing a number of diet-related diseases, from cancer and obesity to constipation and hemorrhoids. This will eventually increase his medical utilization and result in decreased productivity due to being overweight and continued use of tobacco and alcohol.

Failure to include regular exercise as part of the treatment of his hypertension and stress leads to suboptimal physical fitness. Episodic attempts at exercise or recreational activity increase his risk of exercise-induced heart disease and musculoskeletal problems from irregular exertion.

Failure to adequately and proactively address this person's alcohol use results in continuation of a direct cause of his hypertension and may result in progression to alcoholism. At fifteen to seventeen years in his career, the patient's problem with alcohol becomes overtly manifest through work difficulties, family abuse, DWIs, or accidents. This results in a retroactive alcohol rehabilitation program with unknown long-term success. Costs to the company range from $2,500 to over $7,500 for a residential program. At this point, attempts to address some of the underlying causes of this patient's problems, causes that have been ignored yet present from early in his career, may be difficult and unsuccessful. This assumes the patient does not have a serious alcohol-related accident at some point resulting in long-term disability or the need for institutionalized care that further drains medical and community resources.

After retirement, the patient develops angina and is discovered to have coronary artery disease. He is given a potent message by the cardiologist to stop smoking and told to cut the fat in his diet to 30 percent but still does not get specific training, with his wife, on exactly how to do this. He is treated with anti-anginal medications. Cost of these medications averages $1,800 per year or $36,000 for life, assuming he lives for twenty more years. Alternatively, or at a later time, the patient receives a coronary artery bypass graft at a cost of $30,000. This is also a temporary solution as such grafting will likely re-occlude in five to ten years if the contributory causes are not effectively and aggressively addressed.

As any primary care practitioner knows, the above sequence is not uncommon. Patients often display part if not all of these conditions, as well as others, during their lifetimes. Effectively addressing the behavioral roots of this patient's problems is not a simple task nor can it be done by a single individual; a team approach is required. With the level of training and resources currently provided to most physicians, it is not surprising that they often become discouraged when addressing the behavioral causes of these chronic conditions.

Total cost of medications over the lifetime of this patient approaches $140,000. An intensive team approach to lifestyle change and maintenance would cost from $2,500 to $5,000 per individual. This is only 2 to 4 percent of the medication cost alone under the current system. Retroactive "post facto" treatment of chronic disease, the etiologies of which are present from early in the patient's life, will result in continued escalation of the cost of medical care. Early identification and behavioral intervention are the only hope of long-term cost containment, short of reducing the availability of medical treatment when needed.

Medical utilization for lifestyle-related disease represents the tip of the iceberg for those who have low personal resources and who develop disease and dysfunction under routine, life situations. Increased stresses of mobility, job insecurity or dissatisfaction, family difficulties, and so forth will bring into the health care delivery system those individuals whose low level of personal resources and lack of self-care skills are hidden or ignored because they do not use medical services until a crisis presents or because current medical approaches do not address the causes of their dysfunction. Without addressing the issue of chronic disease and dysfunction in a *proactive* manner, the health care system will not be able to enhance personal resources and health or increase the number of patients who function at an optimal level.

Tom Whitmarsh

The Nature of Evidence in Complementary and Alternative Medicine: Ideas from Trials of Homeopathy in Chronic Headache

The emerging field of evidence-based medicine (EBM) has brought to the fore many anomalies within the practice of medicine in general. It has often been commented that the majority of medical interventions have no acceptable scientific evidence base (in the EBM sense),[1] although this assertion has been challenged.[2] Most medical practice is seen to have been based on anecdote and the experience of the individual practitioner of previous cases in which a particular approach was successful for the problem presented.

The research tool that has been developed to provide a more objective basis for medical practice is the randomized, controlled clinical trial (RCT). The RCT is a study in which people are allocated at random to receive one of multiple clinical interventions. One of the patient groups often receives placebo, with which the "active" clinical intervention can be compared at the end of the study. Judgments can then be made about the efficacy or otherwise of the active intervention in that particular clinical situation. The purpose of randomization is to minimize inevitable and unpredictable baseline differences in characteristics between the groups, with the object of lessening bias in the results and thus making the conclusion more believable and robust. The chance of bias can be further lessened by blinding the subjects and the investigators to knowledge of which group the subjects have been randomized to. Full discussion is available elsewhere.[3]

The relatively new science of meta-analysis is held to offer promise within the EBM movement of improving objectivity in clinical medicine. Meta-analysis involves combining the results of many controlled trials (and therefore from many patients) into one outcome statistic to give an apparently definitive answer to the clinical question at hand.

Within the field of complementary and alternative medicine (CAM), too, there are calls for ultimately evidence-based practice.[4] The same tools and criteria should apparently be used to decide if a complementary practice should be considered as a viable treatment for a particular health problem. By implication, those therapies that do not (or cannot) come up to these criteria should not be funded or recommended, and, ethically, patients should in fact be actively discouraged from seeking help along these "disproven" lines.

It is my view that EBM as currently formulated will never be able to inform all medical interventions completely.[5] There is a subjective element in doctor-patient relationships that is part of its essence and will always override the objective, evidence-based approach. Clinicians on the whole will tend to continue to rely on personal or peer group experience, not at the expense of evidence from RCTs, but often on a par with it, according to the individual need(s) they perceive in the suffering person before them.

In this chapter I suggest that the use of complementary therapies and in particular homeopathy should be judged according to the same criteria as are daily used for the practice of medicine in general in the real world. It seems to me that, far from being based on truly different evidence platforms, much of the practice taking place in both conventional and complementary medicine is justifiable in remarkably similar ways. I also want to point to potentially fruitful research directions based on experience in this area and ways in which the existing evidence can be read more thoroughly than has so far been the case.

Thus, one goal is to look at CAM practice from a conventional angle and acknowledge that practices are not really so very different. Another is to view CAM research and practice from within and point out some of the problems, failings, and quality issues that surround CAM research and that can be improved. I will use the example of research in the prophylaxis of migraine and other chronic headache with homeopathy.

Homeopathy and Evidence

Homeopathy aims to stimulate the body's own self-healing powers. It uses preparations often in very small amounts, based on the concept that "like can cure like." In other words, the substance used to promote healing in a sick person would produce a similar clinical picture if given to a healthy person. This is not unlike the process of vaccination, where a tiny amount of inactivated virus is used to provide an appropriate immune response when the body is challenged with that infection.

Homeopathy offers a whole-person approach and aims to embrace many aspects of a person's life. Treatment is therefore very individualistic, and patients with the same conventional medical diagnosis do not necessarily receive the same remedy. Homeopathy has been formulated as a method of treatment and practiced for at least two hundred years in a large number of countries across the world. The concept of treatment by similars and the use of tiny amounts (often in submolecular concentrations) are the two main sticking points in the acceptance of this form of therapy by conventionally trained physicians. Despite this, homeopathy is an accepted part of the state-run health care systems in many countries. For example, there are five homeopathic hospitals in the United Kingdom run by the National Health Service, and homeopathy is an integral part of the national health care systems of India and Brazil. It is reimbursed by state insurance plans in several European countries, including France and Germany. Two hundred years is generally long enough for a completely ineffective form of therapy naturally to fall out of use.[6] In reality, the use of homeopathy is becoming ever more widespread.[7]

Treatment with homeopathy is extremely contentious in conventional medical circles, mainly because it is frankly unbelievable in accepted scientific terms. Is there any evidence of clinical effectiveness that meets conventional scientific standards of evidence? It sometimes comes as a surprise to discover there have been quite a number of randomized and/or double-blind, placebo-controlled trials using clinical homeopathy. These have been collected into systematic reviews and meta-analyses on three occasions in recent years, and the most complete of these is that of Linde.[8]

In Linde's study, the authors tested the hypothesis that the effects seen with homeopathic remedies are equivalent to those seen with placebo. Out of 189 randomized and/or double-blind, placebo-controlled trials identified by diligent searching, 119 met the entry criteria and 89 had adequate data for meta-analysis. An odds ratio was determined for each trial and these were combined to give a single figure, which reflects efficacy. An odds ratio greater than unity (1) indicates greater efficacy of homeopathy than placebo, and the combined odds ratio for the 89 studies was 2.45 (95 percent confidence interval 2.05–2.93). Despite corrections for study quality (a subgroup of the highest-quality studies was analyzed separately) and for possible publication bias, the authors still concluded that there is no evidence that the clinical effects of homeopathy are completely due to placebo. The result is consistent with those of a systematic review in 1991[9] as well as another meta-analysis, which used a different technique for combining p values from the Homeopathic Medicine Research Group of the European Community.[10]

The Linde paper makes a number of very relevant points. Most important, although the overall result of the meta-analysis supported an effect of homeopathy above that of placebo, Linde found very little evidence of reproducibility of results. That is, there are very few conditions in which homeopathy has been tested in rigorous trials on different populations by different research groups. This fact naturally reduces the impact of any positive studies and leads to the author's comment that "there is insufficient evidence from these studies that homeopathic treatment is clearly effective in any one clinical condition." It should be noted that doubts were expressed about the value of the results of Linde's work from the very beginning. Editorials in the same issue of the *Lancet* espoused the view that trials should not be done at all in homeopathy because it cannot possibly be effective.[11]

Nevertheless, homeopathy continues to be used as the treatment of choice in certain situations by well-trained physicians. For example, it is one among many options, both conventional and complementary, for the treatment of chronic headache.[12] The literature is replete with thousands of examples of difficult to manage clinical problems from general internal medicine, pediatrics, dermatology, and psychiatry (among others), where homeopathy has been used to extremely beneficial or even curative effect.[13] It seems, then, that the kind of evidence collected in the Linde meta-analysis (randomized, placebo-controlled trials) does not convince enough to overturn the results of experience of treating individuals who were suffering and no longer suffer as a result of intervention using homeopathy, even among trained physicians. On the one hand, randomized controlled trials of complementary therapies that are negative tend to convince the skeptical conventional physician of ineffectiveness.[14] On the other hand, it seems that positive randomized controlled trials or analyses in complementary therapies do not seem to convince of anything and generate much adverse comment in the conventional medical world.[15]

What might convince skeptics that homeopathy has an action above placebo and brings about useful improvements in health? What would convince "believers" that it does not? The experience of randomized controlled trials of homeopathy in the prophylaxis of migraine and chronic headache conditions offers some pointers that might be helpful in answering these questions. I will come to these later, but first I will discuss conventional management of migraine and the evidence available for practices in current use.

Migraine and Prophylaxis

Migraine is a form of intermittent headache that is present and common in most populations, with a lifetime prevalence of about 15 percent in women and 6 percent in men.[16] It is associated with many symptoms other than headache and causes considerable distress and dysfunction. Many studies have reported substantial loss of workdays due to migraine. For example, one estimate of the cost of lost productivity for employees working outside the home in the United States due to migraine was $1.4 billion per year.[17]

Since a hallmark of the condition is complete freedom from symptoms between attacks, most migraine sufferers treat their attacks with painkilling drugs only when they need them. Simple, easily available painkillers and antiemetics help many sufferers. Recently, a class of drugs was introduced that is very specifically targeted at the pain and other symptoms of migraine (the triptans). Even in the most optimistic studies, however, the efficacy of these agents does not approach 100 percent. There is also a significant number of sufferers who do not respond to acute treatment, or who only have partial response and so are still significantly disabled by their attacks. Others cannot tolerate the side effects of the drugs currently available, or cannot use these drugs in every attack because their attack frequency raises safety concerns about using them too often.

Another approach is to use daily, continual dosing with drugs that are held to act as prophylactics. They cut down the number of acute attacks experienced and thus the amount of acute medication necessary. Initiation of a prophylactic agent has conventionally been considered when two or more attacks are occurring monthly, although with the introduction of the triptans this has risen to around four per month. These are only rough guides, and the real criteria for commencing on a daily prophylactic drug are based on the distress of the individual and how disabling to normal life the attacks are perceived to be. Some people find that one severe, perhaps four-day attack that removes them from their occupation for this length of time each month is worth trying to avoid at any cost, even that of side effects from a drug taken daily. Others are relatively untroubled by four attacks per month, which they treat adequately for their commitments with some over-the-counter analgesia from the pharmacist. It all depends on severity and context.

How effective is conventional drug prophylaxis for migraine? A number of reviews have pointed out that the drugs available for prophylaxis of migraine are not particularly effective when judged by generally accepted criteria.[18] There are also many inconsistencies in the use of these agents by physicians. One survey questioned one hundred U.S. neurologists and ninety-six primary care physicians (PCPs), selected on the basis of their experience in treating a large number of migraine patients.[19] They were asked what their first and second choices of migraine prophylactic therapies were. Top of the list for both groups of physicians was the beta-blocker group of drugs (and propranolol in particular), with about 40 percent using them first line. Tricyclic antidepressants, mainly amitriptyline (neurologists 30 percent, PCPs 15 percent), and calcium channel blockers, mainly verapamil (18 percent and 16 percent, respectively), ranked second and third in both groups. Smaller but significant numbers of physicians used some other drugs as first or second line agents. For example, 13 percent of PCPs reported using a selective serotonin reuptake blocker (SSRI) as prophylaxis.

To test for a correlation between use and efficacy, the authors also performed a review of all published (in English) double-blind, randomized, placebo-controlled trials of prophylaxis of migraine with drugs. They looked at their effect compared with that of placebo and they rated each trial on a five-point scale of scientific rigor (scientific score, ss) as a way of assessing how believable the trial results were (1 = low, 5 = good, with corresponding negative values for trials that showed no benefit over placebo). The three most commonly chosen migraine prophylactics scored very poorly on efficacy and/or study quality parameters. Efficacy is usually defined as a reduction of at least 50 percent in attack frequency.[20] The review suggests that this may not be particularly satisfactory to the patient who develops four or more severe and disabling migraine attacks per month.

Only one study out of all those of the top three drugs, of propranolol, suggested a benefit of more than 50 percent over placebo, and this had a very low score of scientific rigor (ss = 1). Sixteen out of the eighteen trials of propranolol did suggest some benefit over placebo, with propranolol reducing headache frequency by 10 to 76 percent (mean $\pm$ SD = 33 $\pm$ 19) relative to placebo. The average ss, however, was poor (1.44, range −4 to 5). The trial with the highest ss showed a 31 percent

improvement over placebo, but the trial with the next best score
(ss = −4) demonstrated no benefit over placebo. There are many fewer
studies of amitriptyline and verapamil, but conclusions are broadly
similar.

It would seem that the results of these trials are at least conflicting,
and at worst misleading. An especially surprising result was the preference expressed by 13 percent of PCPs for SSRIs as first or second
choice for migraine prophylaxis. There is no justification from the trials
for this, with just two studies, one showing some benefit over placebo
(ss = 3) and the other failing to (ss = 2). This represents a large number
of headache sufferers and millions of dollars spent on agents that have
not been shown to prevent migraine. The authors conclude that "most
reported trials of migraine preventative drugs have doubtful scientific
merit and have been poorly reported. Also, an agent that provides more
than 50 percent improvement in migraine headache frequency is still
awaited. Accordingly, physician's choice of anti-migraine drugs remains
largely empiric."

Homeopathy and Migraine Prophylaxis

The earliest double-blind RCT in this area was that of Brigo.[21] He
assigned thirty patients to active homeopathic treatment and thirty to
placebo and followed them for four months. He demonstrated highly
significant and very clinically relevant reductions in all parameters of
headache, including frequency, severity, and consumption of analgesia.

Soon after the Linde meta-analysis was published,[22] three more
clinical trials of homeopathy in chronic headache became available,
providing a potential example of replication. It is these I want to
concentrate on, using the whole series to demonstrate problems practically encountered, to show how inappropriately designed and performed
trials can misrepresent a therapy, and to try to see what lessons for
future research there are in these trials.

The trials are summarized in a table from a second review that
Linde performed of trials of individualized homeopathy (as opposed to
other forms).[23] Elsewhere in his analysis, Linde used two different scales
of methodological quality to rate the trials. All four headache trials
were apparently well performed, being rated as either "likely to have
good methodological quality" or to be "unlikely to have major flaws."
The three 1997 trials were really attempts to confirm the startlingly
positive results that Brigo apparently achieved in the 1991 study. In
particular, the study with which I was involved set out specifically to

replicate Brigo's results, using up-to-the-minute migraine diagnostic criteria and trial design. I was trying to understand why, if homeopathy is as useful a treatment as homeopaths claim,[24] very little evidence of reproducibility has been demonstrated from such well-designed trials.

At face value, only Brigo's study shows homeopathy to be anything other than equivalent to placebo. I would suggest, however, that the conclusion that homeopathy is not effective in migraine and chronic headache can be reasonably challenged as erroneous if the trials are considered in greater detail and the concentration on conventional measures of outcome less strict. In any case, there are potential difficulties in interpretation of all these trial results, and I will now describe some of these.

Straumsheim and colleagues studied seventy-three patients with migraine, diagnosed according to standard criteria of the International Headache Society (IHS),[25] of whom sixty-eight completed the study.[26] They were randomized to individualized homeopathic treatment (thirty-five patients) or identical placebo (thirty-three patients). A baseline month was used to record clinical data, and then treatment was undertaken for four months, using daily diary cards as the measure of migraine attack frequency, intensity, and analgesic consumption. Results from the diary card analysis reveal a reduction of about 30 percent in migraine frequency over the time of the trial, with no significant difference between the active and placebo groups. Migraine attack frequency is conventionally the recommended primary measure of outcome in migraine prophylaxis trials.[27] Results were similar for mean pain intensity and analgesic consumption.

Another measure of effectiveness was also used. The patients were diagnosed and suggested for entry into the trial by an independent neurologist, who also assessed with the patients their perception of the outcome of the trial after four months. This assessment shows a significant difference in attack frequency per month in favor of the active homeopathy group (p = 0.04). The authors justifiably conclude that homeopathic prophylaxis of migraine was not shown to be inactive by all measures. A more patient-focused assessment than simply counting the number of attacks produced a result in favor of homeopathy.

In another study, my colleagues and I randomized sixty-three migraine patients, again diagnosed by IHS criteria, to receive either homeopathy or placebo, with a one-month placebo run-in for all patients.[28] Treatment was for three months and diary entries logged attack frequency, with measures of intensity and analgesic consumption as secondary outcome measures. The attack frequency declined slightly in both groups, 19 percent in the active group and 16 percent in the placebo group, which is nonsignificant over the course of the trial. Unfortunately, there was a chance difference at baseline between the groups both for primary outcome measure and for headache severity.

The placebo group had significantly more frequent but less severe headaches. Closer analysis revealed that the homeopathy group lost their moderate to severe headaches, whereas the placebo group lost their mild headaches only. In addition, the course of change was different in the two groups. Improvement occurred early in the placebo group, followed by a return toward baseline by the end of the trial. By contrast, the active group improved later in the trial and was continuing to improve as the trial finished. Thus the attack frequency was relatively stable over the short treatment period, but the headache severity may have changed significantly, which is possibly more relevant to patients.

The pattern of change suggests that, had the trial gone on longer, the two groups would have separated and a significant difference between active and placebo would have been shown. Furthermore, an analysis of a measure of patient assessment of efficacy (not reported in the original paper) favors homeopathy significantly. Had such a measure been chosen as a primary outcome measure, the trial would have been regarded as positive for homeopathy. We regretted various flaws in the design of this trial, such as the chance disparity at entry that could have been avoided with stratification of the randomization code according to headache frequency and also that the trial period, chosen according to IHS recommendations, was not longer.

A third trial of homeopathy in chronic headache was reported by Walach.[29] Ninety-eight patients were entered, and, by chance, sixty-one were randomized to receive active homeopathy and only thirty-seven placebo. The population was not restricted to migraine, with the other major diagnosis being tension-type headache. There was a six-week baseline run-in and then twelve weeks of treatment. The last four weeks of the baseline were compared with the last four weeks of treatment in terms of headache frequency, intensity (assessed on a visual analog scale), and analgesic consumption.

There was a little improvement in both groups, with no significant differences in any measure of outcome. For example, the frequency of headache was reduced by one headache-day in four weeks and the mean duration of headache was only twenty-two minutes less per day. This is convincingly negative for homeopathy. However, the patients were a very difficult group to help by any standards. They had a median headache duration of eight hours per day and the median headache history was twenty-three years.

The prescribing method was chosen to try to maximize the likelihood of success with homeopathy. Six homeopathic doctors were available for consultation. Each case was taken by one of them and discussed with the other five before prescribing. The first interview lasted for a mean of 156 minutes. This method of prescribing (by consensus, it would seem) and the very long first interview do not correspond to the usual practice of most homeopathic physicians. There is no evidence, for example, of whether six heads are better than one in homeopathic prescribing. Some homeopaths would see this method as over-controlled and likely to downgrade the prescribers' intuitive response to the patient, thus actually reducing the efficacy of homeopathy.

The Need for Careful Analysis

A systematic review of the four migraine trials concluded that the trial data to date do not suggest that homeopathy is effective in the prophylaxis of migraine beyond a placebo effect.[30] Given other conditions, other designs, more typical patient populations, and more patient-centered outcome measures as primary measures of efficacy, it is likely that at least Straumsheim's and my studies would have proved more favorable to homeopathy. When patient assessment of efficacy (my study) or assessment of some kind of global improvement by the patient with the neurologist (Straumsheim's) are used as measures of efficacy, then more positive results emerge.

Careful reading of the literature is very important. The headline message of all three attempted repetitions of the initial, extremely successful trial of homeopathy in migraine prophylaxis was that it is ineffective. Looking more closely, though, it is possible to see how different all the trials are with their confounding factors, and that buried in all the noise there are some more positive messages. Indeed, the author of the review concludes by saying "due to several caveats (e.g., paucity of RCTs) it seems premature to make final judgment on this matter."

Trial results (complementary or conventional) should not be believed without careful analysis. Only then is it possible to avoid false conclusions based on flimsy premises, which in the relatively small field of CAM research (especially homeopathy) can have a large and devastating impact (for example, on continued funding). I have often heard that exceptional claims require exceptional evidence. As the evidence apparently needs to be more robust to enable conventional belief in nonconventional therapies, so the scrutiny of the evidence needs to be very strong and careful.

From this sort of analysis I conclude that only the trial of Walach is truly negative, and this is explicable on the grounds of having such difficult patients to help and a very unusual method of prescribing. Therefore, instead of only one positive trial in four, we have only one truly negative trial in four. Things are not as black as they have been painted.[31] This looks a lot more hopeful and begins to compare favorably with the trial base for conventional prescribing, especially if the substantially lower financial and infrastructural support available for research in homeopathy is taken into consideration.

In comparing conventional prophylaxis using the most commonly chosen drugs with homeopathic prophylaxis of migraine, the overall evidence of worthwhile migraine relief from high-quality RCTs is not particularly different. It is possible to choose a single trial from either field to support any contention about efficacy or otherwise. It has been said that "the plural of anecdotes is not evidence," yet homeopathic and nonhomeopathic physicians will continue to use empirical methods of prescribing, based on personal experience. Physicians will go on using propranolol (or homeopathy) despite the conflicting messages from the trials because, in their experience, they judge it effective.

Cant and Sharma discuss how doctors justify individual therapeutic acts and how alternative medicine can fit into a general theory of medical knowledge by reference to Pickstone's ideas.[32] Pickstone defines "biographical" medicine as "the medical knowledge derived from the observation of the effects of disease on particular bodies, encountered in the life courses of given individuals." From this point of view, anecdotal evidence may be highly significant. Pickstone contrasts this sort of knowledge with the analytical knowledge of hospital-based medicine, the experimental knowledge of the university laboratory, and "techno-science," usually generated by industrial companies.[33]

How should we be demonstrating this real-world effectiveness (as opposed to merely comparative efficacy over placebo in the rather artificial set-up of RCTs)? I propose that we need a more subtle approach to outcome measures in homeopathic trials and complementary medicine trials in general in order to try to access the less easily defined changes and benefits patients consistently report with homeopathy and other complementary therapies. These could include quality of life, general well-being, and patient satisfaction issues. There needs to be a wider appreciation and availability of outcome scales that can elucidate the less obvious, but significant, information. Ideally, there should be concentrated efforts at designing new, validated, easy-to-use measuring tools that can be widely applied in complementary therapies.

Prospective observational studies would give more robust information than single case experiences and can certainly generate evidence that might be sufficient for changing skeptical opinion of the value of CAM in day-to-day use. Audits of outcome in large series of clinical practice of either single conditions or homeopathy as a whole (or, of course, another complementary therapy) look promising. Successes need to be built on, and active communication between researchers can help avoid pitfalls.

In conclusion, there are two strands to the arguments I have presented. The first is that there is evidence of efficacy above placebo for a particular complementary therapy (homeopathy) in a particular condition (migraine), using standards dictated by conventional methodology and criteria. I have also suggested that many conventional physicians ignore or fail fully to assess the evidence available from RCTs and nonetheless practice very effectively using broadly anecdotal or other empirical criteria, a charge often leveled at practitioners of complementary medicine.

In my own practice as a general physician with expertise in homeopathy, I embrace research results from all areas of inquiry, complementary and conventional. The less tangible aspects of the practice of medicine and the doctor-patient relationship, though, are usually in the foreground. On the whole, this is the position of most physicians.[34] In the practice of medicine, two apparent extremes, conventional and complementary, in fact approach each other. Future research in complementary medicine should build on this common ground of clinical concerns, using new methods and measures of outcome to demonstrate effectiveness. This holds the promise of ultimately improving patient care, improving the effectiveness of the therapies, and justifying continued and expanding funding for complementary medicine.

NOTES

1. Richard Smith, "Where Is the Wisdom . . . ? The Poverty of Medical Evidence," *British Medical Journal* 303 (October 5, 1991): 798–99.

2. Jonathan Ellis et al., "Inpatient Medicine is Evidence-Based," *Lancet* 346 (August 12, 1995): 407–10; P. Gill et al., "Evidence-Based General Practice: A Retrospective Study of Interventions in One Training Practice," *British Medical Journal* 312 (March 30, 1996): 819–21.

3. Alejandro Jadad, *Randomised Controlled Trials: A User's Guide* (London: BMJ Books, 1998).

4. M. Angell and J. P. Kassiver, "Alternative Medicine: The Risks of Untested and Unregulated Remedies," *NEJM* 339, no. 12 (1998): 839–41.

5. Trisha Greenhalgh, "Narrative-Based Medicine in an Evidence-Based World," *British Medical Journal* 318 (January 30, 1999): 323–25.

6. Harald Walach, "Methodology Beyond Clinical Trials," in *Homeopathy: A Critical Appraisal*, ed. Edzard Ernst and Eckhart G. Hahn (Oxford: Butterworth–Heinemann, 1998), p. 49.

7. Peter Fisher and Adam Ward, "Complementary Medicine in Europe," *British Medical Journal* 309 (July 9, 1994): 107–11.

8. Jos Kleijnen, Paul Knipschild, and Gerben ter Riet, "Clinical Trials of Homeopathy," *British Medical Journal* 302 (February 9, 1991): 316–23; Klaus Linde et al., "Are the Clinical Effects of Homeopathy Placebo Effects? A Meta-analysis of Placebo-controlled Trials," *Lancet* 350 (September 20, 1997): 834–43; M. Cucherat et al., "Evidence of Clinical Efficacy of Homeopathy: A Meta-analysis of Clinical Trials," *European Journal of Clinical Pharmacology* 56, no. 1 (2000): 27–33.

9. Kleijnen, Knipschild, and Riet, "Clinical Trials of Homeopathy."

10. Cucherat et al., "Evidence of Clinical Efficacy of Homeopathy."

11. Jan P. Vandenbroucke, "Homeopathy Trials: Going Nowhere," *Lancet* 350 (September 20, 1997): 824.

12. Thomas E. Whitmarsh, "The Place and Efficacy of Complementary Therapies," in *The Effective Management of Headache,* ed. Peter J. Goadsby, Andrew J. Dowson, and Andrew Miles (London: Aesculapius Medical Press, 1999), pp. 135–54.

13. For some examples, see issues of *British Homeopathic Journal* (1911–present); *Proceedings of the Professional Case Conferences of the American Institute of Homeopathy* (Edmonds, Wash.: International Foundation for Homeopathy, 1989–1996); and *Homeopathic Links* (1987–present).

14. W. D. Gerber, "Classical Homeopathic Treatment," editorial commentary, *Cephalalgia* 17, no. 2 (1997): 101.

15. See the correspondence following a well-performed trial in homeopathy, *Lancet* (November 8, 1986): 1106–07. The trial was David Reilly et al., "Is Homeopathy a Placebo Response? Controlled Trial of Homeopathic Potency, with Pollen in Hayfever as Model," *Lancet* (October 18, 1986): 881–85.

16. B. K. Rasmussen et al., "Epidemiology of Headache in a General Population: A Prevalence Study," *Journal of Clinical Epidemiology* 44, no. 11 (1991): 1147–57.

17. Kim Price, "The Epidemiology and Economics of Headache," in *The Effective Management of Headache*, pp. 3–22.

18. Nabih M. Ramadan, L. L. Schultz, and S. J. Gilkey, "Migraine Prophylactic Drugs: Proof of Efficacy, Utilization and Cost," *Cephalalgia* 17, no. 2 (1997): 73–80; Andrew J. Dowson, "Treatment of Headache and Prophylaxis," in *The Effective Management of Headache*, pp. 63–76.

19. Ramadan, Schultz, and Gilkey, "Migraine Prophylactic Drugs."

20. David Bates et al., *Migraine Management Guidelines: A Strategy for the Modern Management of Migraine* (London: Synergy Medical Education, 1997).

21. Bruno Brigo and Giovanni Serpelloni, "Homeopathic Treatment of Migraine: A Randomized, Double-Blind Controlled Study of Sixty Cases (Homeopathy Versus Placebo)," *Berlin Journal on Research in Homeopathy* 1, no. 2 (1991): 98–106.

22. Linde et al., "Are the Clinical Effects of Homeopathy Placebo Effects?"

23. Klaus Linde and Dieter Melchart, "Randomised Controlled Trials of Individualised Homeopathy: A State-of-the-Art Review," *Journal of Alternative and Complementary Medicine* 4, no. 4 (1998): 371–88.

24. Thomas E. Whitmarsh, "When Conventional Treatment Is Not Enough: A Case of Migraine without Aura Responding to Homeopathy," *Journal of Alternative and Complementary Medicine* 3, no. 2 (1997): 159–62.

25. International Headache Society Classification Committee, "Classification and Diagnostic Criteria for Headache Disorders, Cranial Neuralgias and Facial Pain," *Cephalalgia* 8, Supplement 7 (1988): 13–96.

26. P. A. Straumsheim et al., "Homeopathic Treatment of Migraine: A Double Blind, Placebo Controlled Trial of 68 Patients," *British Homeopathic Journal* 89, no. 1 (2000): 4–7; originally published as P. A. Straumsheim et al., "Homeopatisk Behandling av Migrene: En Dobbelt-Blind, Placebokontrollert Studie av 68 Pasienter," *Dynamis,* no. 2 (1997): 18–21.

27. International Headache Society Committee on Clinical Trials in Migraine, "Guidelines for Controlled Trials of Drugs in Migraine, First edition," *Cephalalgia* 11, no. 1 (1991): 1–12.

28. Thomas E. Whitmarsh, Donna M. Coleston-Shields, and Timothy J. Steiner, "Double-Blind Randomized Placebo-Controlled Study of Homeopathic Prophylaxis of Migraine," *Cephalalgia* 17, no. 5 (1997): 600–604.

29. Harald Walach et al., "Classical Homeopathic Treatment of Chronic Headaches," *Cephalalgia* 17, no. 2 (1997): 119–26.

30. Edzard Ernst, "Homeopathic Prophylaxis of Headaches and Migraine? A Systematic Review," *Journal of Pain and Symptom Management* 18, no. 5 (1999): 353–57.

31. Anon, "No Evidence for Homeopathic Prophylaxis for Migraine," *Bandolier* 7, no. 1 (2000): 5.

32. Sarah Cant and Ursula Sharma, *A New Medical Pluralism? Alternative Medicine, Doctors, Patients and the State* (London: UCL Press, 1999), pp. 99–100.

33. John V. Pickstone, "Ways of Knowing: Towards a Historical Sociology of Science, Technology and Medicine," *British Journal of the History of Science* 26 (1993): 433–58.

34. Greenhalgh, "Narrative-Based Medicine in an Evidence-Based World."

PAUL ROOT WOLPE

Medical Culture and CAM Culture: Science and Ritual in the Academic Medical Center

After a period of wholesale rejection of complementary and alternative medical (CAM) forms, biomedical institutions seem to have begun embracing them wholesale. Academic, private, and community medical centers have been establishing CAM clinics, holding conferences, and advertising alternative, traditional, and spiritually based therapies to their patients. At first glance, such a dramatic turnabout seems puzzling: no new scientific findings are compelling enough to justify bringing these modalities into mainstream practice. Many commentators (including this author) have written that the impetus to establish CAM services lies more in a hospital's marketing department than in its medical director's office. Confronted by economic pressures, and clued in to the power of the CAM market by high-profile articles such as Eisenberg's report in the *New England Journal of Medicine,* administrators perceived a relatively low-cost way to respond to consumer demand.[1]

While there is little doubt that the economics of CAM has had an important role to play in its current incarnation, relying exclusively on such an approach simplifies the deeper resonance biomedicine has with the society in which it operates. All medicine is embedded in cultural context and draws its power from its cultural legitimacy. Medicine reflects its culture in many ways, including its reframing of the disjunctive moment of illness in an explanatory framework that allows the culture to make sense and gives meaning to its suffering. Medicine incorporates a society's most sophisticated technologies, usually supports its most valued "professionals" (think of the shaman in tribal culture), and reflects broad-based religious, political, and economic values and beliefs. Medicine encodes within it definitions of disease and "dis-ease," cultural constructs of dying and death, a sense of life's value ("quality of life"), the cultural role of science, society's relationship to God or other ultimate values, kinship relations, nutritional beliefs, ritual constructs—the list could go on—of a particular society at a particular moment in its history. In other words, medicine is a constantly evolving social product.

Medicine's embedded values are thus suprascientific (as are science's itself). The culture contributes to medicine's values through its mythologies, rituals, base assumptions about life and health, religious beliefs, and lay medical beliefs. While medicine's cultural embeddedness is easy to see when we study premodern cultures, we tend to overvalue science as a means of mitigating cultural influences in our own cultural healing form, "biomedicine." There is a pervasive belief that, for the most part, biomedicine has purged itself of cultural influences by being "scientific" and not mythological. Demonstrations of cultural influence or underpinnings of biomedicine are usually lamented and met with calls for more science, as if fact can drive value from our medicine.

Cultural differences, however, are not due to lack of data. Lynn Payer, for example, has studied the differences in diagnosis and treatment of disease among the United States, France, England, and Germany, and has found in the four, industrialized, high-technology, scientific countries profound and deep differences in their interpretations of disease and their modes of treatment.[2] For example, German diagnostics is dominated by cardiac problems, and Germans take six times the amount of heart drugs per capita as the French or English. The most common cardiac diagnosis in Germany, *Herzinsuffizienz,* does not exist in the other three countries. Payer argues persuasively that the German preoccupation with circulation and other German medical traditions are largely due to the influence of German romanticism, the palette of cultural values from which German medicine is constructed.

While not denying the existence of cultural influences on medicine in general, the response of critics is that such influences can be mitigated by more and better science. The existence of diseases such as *Herzinsuffizienz* can be verified or refuted. Yet this fails to recognize that definitions of disease are about cultural judgments of desirability and function, that medicine derives its definitions of disease from normative judgments that are taken for granted, and that when medicine falls out of step with the culture it serves, it is medicine, not the culture, that generally changes to restore balance.

It is precisely biomedicine's reluctance to recognize the political, social, and even mythological and ritualistic underpinnings of its nature that explains the turnabout in modern medicine's attitude toward CAM.

Biomedicine cannot at the same time defend its hegemony by claiming singular scientific legitimacy and also freely admit that it has an arbitrary and ultimately scientifically narrow view of the body and health, that much of its armamentarium is untested and ritualized, and that it ignores large swaths of what the public feels is crucial to its health—religion, spirituality, subjective experiences, emotional context and reaction, lay theories of etiology and prevention, folk and alternative healing modalities, and so on. Instead, it tries to "scientize" those aspects of health in order to justify pursuing them in the ways its constituency demands. The emergence of CAM thus *is* a marketing phenomenon, but in the most noble sense of that word—it is a way to respond to society's demand to reinvigorate the "art" of medicine, its attention to the subjective, ritualized, and mythological, under the guise of scientific scrutiny.

Definitions of CAM

The culturally constructed nature of medical definitions can clearly be seen in the attempt to define CAM. After years of trying to define CAM by its attributes (e.g., its untested nature, its lay or foreign origins, or its unscientific rationale), it has become clear that the only reasonable definition, insofar as there is one, is political, economic, and social (see Kopelman, this volume). CAM as a category has no internal consistency. What is the definitional rationale for grouping chelation therapy (a sophisticated chemical infusion technique that was fully developed in World War II for heavy metal toxicity and is now touted as a circulatory enhancer), acupuncture (an ancient Chinese healing modality based on energy meridians), and chiropractic (a spinal manipulation technique invented in the 1880s by a magnetic healer in Iowa)? Only their relative estrangement from the idiosyncratic constellation of therapies we equally arbitrarily group under "orthodox medicine."

CAM is what sociologists refer to as a *residual category*. It is defined not by its internal coherence but by its exclusion from other categories of medicine. It is a carve-out category for modalities that do not seem to fit the values of the modern biomedical world view. Medicine has many such categories; they serve to defuse inherent tensions and cope with difficult anomalies. For example, if the biological organism undergoes physiological changes in the absence of a scientific explanation, we call it a "placebo" response; if there are symptoms in the absence of identifiable pathology, we call it "psychosomatic" illness; if there seems to be unexpected spontaneous resolution of a disease or remission of a cancer, we do not take it seriously as a healing event but see it as beyond our understanding because we did not cause it with our medicines. We dismiss these categories as unimportant and uninteresting to our science. (How much of its relative resources does the National Institutes of Health spend on studying the placebo response or psychosomatic illness, or does the National Cancer Institute spend on studying spontaneous remissions, despite the overwhelming evidence that these are some of the most powerful healing forces we know of?) These phenomena are relegated to residual categories that "explain" them, and thus they are no longer seen as anomalous or threatening to our views of medicine. The same strategy has relegated hundreds of dissimilar therapies to one category, "Complementary and Alternative Medicine," where, until recently, they could be conveniently dismissed en masse as quackery or, at best, as an anthropological curiosity.

Science and CAM

In congressional testimony in 1998, Richard Klausner, director of the National Cancer Institute (NCI), said, "Several months ago, as a result of our own concerns and the constructive input from the CAM community, we removed from the NCI web site all previous CAM information and are creating new information that treats CAM dispassionately and fairly."

The search for empirical truths has social and ethical underpinnings. What is considered "a fact" and what is not a fact are judgments based on cultural value, and they help sculpt science itself. Motokawa, in comparing current Japanese and American science, described their fundamental differences partly in terms of how each culture thinks of facts, inspired by deep-seated religious and ideological assumptions.[3] In Western religion, he suggests, there is one God who knows all, is omnipotent, rules over Man, and created the world with a purpose. In Zen Buddhism, there is no creator god, no purpose of creation, no mediators or gap between man and the ultimate. Accordingly, science in the West searches for uniform and universal rules, the "grand unified theory"—the natural product of a single omnipotent creator. Eastern science emphasizes difference and the multiplicity of natural rules, the result of a karmic world where individual transformation is the goal, not unification with the Mind of God. The Western way of thinking links revealed truths to language and text ("first came the Word . . ."), so for a fact to have value it must first be interpreted through words. Facts must be connected to other facts by a framework of linked sets of universal rules ("theories"); an uninterpretable fact is seen as a curiosity and is put in a conceptual holding cell until it can be "understood." In the Eastern way of thinking, in contrast, truth is found through silence and removing the self from mediating the world, and so science is based on *fact* (not interpretation). A single fact, standing alone, is "truth," even in the absence of a theory that "explains" it. Such differences, Motokawa claims, lead to very different scientific methods, different scientific products, and different professional values and routes to advancement—different science.

Even within Western science, how you frame your inquiry, what you consider a worthy observation, and, once produced, how a fact is considered and framed change over time and differ between disciplines. I have tried to show elsewhere the ideologically driven nature of theory choice and theory reception in modern institutionalized science, which follows a long tradition in the sociology of science in showing the social and cultural influences on scientific theory formation and interpretation.[4] Though studies in the sociology, history, and philosophy of science have shown repeatedly that science is, to a large degree, a cultural and social pursuit, too often in the CAM discussion science itself is rendered unproblematic. CAM opponents argue that CAM supporters are "antiscience" or do not recognize the legitimacy of exploring CAM scientifically. Yet, as Richard Klausner suggests in the quote above, science is not just science, and facts are not just facts. The change in orthodox medicine's approach to CAM is not due to new facts, but new values.

Serious CAM advocates are not antiscience and do not advocate abandoning empirical study (if they can get funded and get their studies into medical journals). The argument is not over science or no science, but *which* science. Those entrenched in a particular set of cultural approaches to science have had difficulty in understanding that it is not *science* that many CAM supporters have rejected but a set of values that predisposed *this particular form* of science to dismiss CAM as a serious healing modality a priori. Biomedicine's tendency to slight the role of subjective illness experiences in physical healing, its tendency to dismiss the value of subjective experience as a "fact" worthy of attention, has differentiated it from a host of healing forms that regard such information as vitally important, and from a scientific world view that does not dismiss the impact of such factors as epiphenomenal. The emergence of CAM in academic medicine has thus challenged biomedical science to reexamine its values and to alter them, if only slightly. That is an accomplishment of no little merit.

As CAM enters the academic medical center, researchers who take it seriously will be forced to challenge existing standards of scientific inquiry. To assess CAM reliably, researchers will have to ask a variety of questions. What is the role of subjective assessments of improvement? What is considered a good outcome in this therapy, and are good outcomes in general merely relative to the goals of the practitioner and client? What do we *really* mean by a placebo response, and how should we evaluate therapies that are linked to their context and do not do well stripped down and applied mechanically? How do we evaluate a modality tied to a practitioner, where the care and concern of the practitioner are an important part of the modality itself? How do we assess spirituality, care, concern, emotional context, and other relationship variables when they are seen as an integral part of a therapy, not as, at best, a supportive add-on as the bioactive mechanism operates? How do we evaluate therapies that categorize patients differently, or that suggest that each patient must be considered as an individual, thus rendering the grouping of patients into subpopulations impossible? The irony of the recent change in the attitude of the medical establishment, thinking they would assimilate CAM quickly and easily, is that CAM's presence may in fact pose a challenge to some of medicine's comfortable scientific assumptions.

CAM in the Academic Medical Center

Medical institutions throughout the country have begun to incorporate CAM. Yet, perhaps ironically, the same underlying misunderstanding of the relationship of culture to medicine that resulted in the premature and unfair rejection of CAM in the past has now led to an unreflective, wholesale acceptance of CAM. Because medicine tends to be blind to the mythological, ritualized, and culturally embedded aspects of its philosophy and praxis, it generally denies the role these dynamics play in healing. It therefore believes that if it dispenses with the competing rituals and cultural dynamics of CAM, it will not make any difference. Most medical centers assume that importing CAM into the clinic is in no fundamental sense different than establishing a new rehabilitation service or physical therapy clinic, that it will simply be another billed service in the conventional medical system.

The conventionalization of CAM in the academic medical center is part of a long history of medicine gaining control over modalities by co-opting them. The establishment of CAM services is predicated on (1) the capacity to integrate these services without disrupting or challenging the existing system, (2) the ability of physicians and administrators to retain control over the modalities, and (3) their profitability. The work of Eisenberg and his colleagues has framed the presentation of CAM in terms of the need, and even the obligation, of physicians to acknowledge, discuss, and eventually take control of their patients' use of CAM.[5] The National Center for Complementary and Alternative Medicine is establishing itself as the arbiter of the efficacy of these modalities through its rapidly increasing research budget. Major medical journals are now publishing CAM research—some of it even demonstrating positive results—and national conferences on CAM, sponsored by academic institutions, have become commonplace. Centers for integrated medicine, CAM research centers, and courses in CAM for medical students and residents are germinating throughout the country. In March 2000, the president of the United States issued an executive order to establish a Commission on Complementary and Alternative Medicine Policy.

The rush to co-opt a previously rejected modality, to remove it from its community or ethnic moorings and reassign it to the academic medical center, is not a new phenomenon in medicine. American medicine has a history of delegitimizing lay healers and then assimilating their knowledge.[6] What is happening now was foreshadowed by the reaction to acupuncture in the early 1970s, when physicians tried to assert dominance over a healing form about which they knew little and cared even less until it was shown that it was desired by consumers and potentially profitable.[7] Once academic medical centers were convinced that CAM was profitable (either in and of itself or as a value-added service to lure consumers to higher-profit medical services) and that it was feasible to offer it without compromising their scientific mission, what had been dismissed as quackery became worthy of serious scientific scrutiny. Yet those who rushed to incorporate CAM may have underestimated its potential for changing the academic medical center itself.

CAM is attractive to its consumers in part because of the relationship with the healer that it fosters, the sense of personal responsibility it engages, and the cultural and ritualized environment in which it is offered. It may prove to be difficult to duplicate that interaction in medical institutions. Some CAM practitioners will not want to enter an academic medical center because it means relinquishing autonomy and practicing a different kind of healing than they are accustomed to.

Some patients will not want to receive services there for the same reason. Many academic medical centers may quickly find that CAM is not the easily assimilated, consumer-friendly service they had counted on because it is precisely its cultural assumptions that they cannot maintain.

CAM's Challenge to Orthodox Medicine

The ethical challenges of CAM are not only the ones often cited, such as determining efficacy, licensing and credentialing, and overcoming resistance from old-school physicians. There is a deeper question of the challenge that CAM poses to hospitals' institutional culture, to their basic assumptions about provision of care, to their mission, and to their philosophy of medicine. It is therefore likely that many of the efforts to establish CAM services will eventually fail. The CAM they import will be stripped of the very ritual and therapeutic philosophy that made it attractive to many patients in the first place. And medical centers that find success with CAM because they are attentive to the cultural, political, and social context in which it is offered may paradoxically find themselves transformed by the presence of CAM services.

As the experiment of CAM integration continues, the ethical challenge it will present may be to the entire edifice of orthodox medicine. The medical philosophy of many CAM modalities, their therapeutics, and the practitioners that employ them all present a cultural challenge to the underlying assumptions that support scientific medicine. People are attracted to CAM for many reasons, including the belief that it is efficacious. But the rise of alternative medicine over the past few decades was due as much to its cultural symbolism and philosophical framework as to its healing potential. In a time of stuffy, close-minded medical thinking, "going alternative" was symbolic of the rejection of establishment medicine, a countercultural political display akin to bra-burning or wearing a pink triangle. It is yet to be seen whether institutionalized CAM will eventually disappear as its cachet wears off, or whether its ideological challenge to biomedical assumptions changes the very system it was meant to enrich.

NOTES

1. David M. Eisenberg et al., "Unconventional Medicine in the United States: Prevalence, Costs, and Patterns of Use," *NEJM* 328, no. 4 (1993): 246–52.

2. Lynn Payer, *Medicine and Culture: Varieties of Treatments in the United States, England, West Germany, and France* (London: Penguin Books, 1988).

3. T. Motokawa, "Sushi Science and Hamburger Science," *Perspectives in Biology and Medicine* 32, no. 4 (1989): 489–504.

4. Paul Root Wolpe, "The Dynamics of Heresy in a Profession," *Social Science and Medicine* 39, no. 9 (1994): 1133–48; Robert K. Merton, *The Sociology of Science: Theoretical and Empirical Investigations* (Chicago: University of Chicago Press, 1973); Paul Root Wolpe, "The Holistic Heresy: Strategies of Ideological Control in the Medical Profession," *Social Science and Medicine* 31, no. 8 (1990): 913–23.

5. D. M. Eisenberg, "Advising Patients Who Seek Alternative Medical Therapies," *Annals of Internal Medicine* 127, no. 1 (1997): 61–69; D. M. Eisenberg et al., "Trends in Alternative Medicine Use in the United States, 1990–1997: Results of a Follow-up National Survey," *JAMA* 280, no. 18 (1998): 1569–75; M. S. Wetzel, D. M. Eisenberg, and T. J. Kaptchuk, "Courses Involving Complementary and Alternative Medicine at US Medical Schools," *JAMA* 280, no. 9 (1998): 784–87.

6. Paul Starr, *The Social Transformation of American Medicine: The Rise of a Sovereign Profession and the Making of a Vast Industry* (New York: Basic Books, 1982).

7. Paul Root Wolpe, "The Maintenance of Professional Authority: Acupuncture and the American Physician," *Social Problems* 32 (June 1985): 409–24.

ALFRED I. TAUBER

The Quest for Holism in Medicine

When David Eisenberg finally told the secret about the appeal of complementary and alternative medicine (CAM) in America, it sent shock waves through the biomedical establishment.[1] Conventional medicine had enjoyed a hegemony since World War II that suddenly appeared to be in jeopardy. Its sanctimonious authority was being disputed not within the medical schools or clinical journals, and not even in Congress, but through the persistent walking of patients to other kinds of practitioners. This social revolt has gained increasing attention through the 1990s, and this collection of essays acutely reflects the legitimate basis for a fair hearing of the alternative challenge. The discussion of the nature and place of so-called complementary medicine relative to conventional medicine has no readily accepted structure, and consequently this collection reflects the various agendas underfoot.

Given the various ways we might approach the general question, I see three issues dominating the discussion about CAM. The first is a "local" problem: the need for data and criteria for evaluation of so-called nonorthodox therapies. This is hardly a minor challenge, but in many ways it is the most accessible. Such issues as the design of clinical trials, the assessment of the placebo effect, and the need for appropriate clinical response criteria all fall under this category. The second matter is to unpack the implications of the challenge to conventional medicine. To the extent that alternative therapies are regarded as contesting the sanctity of scientific-based clinical medicine, the struggle between "orthodoxy" and "alternatives" has far-reaching repercussions. Putting aside the semantic difficulties of defining each camp, I am referring to how "conventional" medicine might adjust to public demands and admit certain kinds of therapies that both originate outside scientific biomedicine and have, as yet, no scientific basis for adoption. What are the politico-economic and ideological implications of such an accommodation, if one is even possible to negotiate?

The third area of discussion concerns defining *what*, indeed, is being debated under the rubric of "alternative medicine." Looking at these essays in a broad historical and philosophical context, I believe we are witnessing only the latest chapter in an ongoing debate that dates back to the nineteenth century concerning the reductive versus holistic basis of medicine. This struggle appears in various guises, some pertaining to different epistemological strategies—for example, the dominating role of positivism as opposed to other modes of knowing—and others having even broader cultural and historical roots that reflect differing visions of the individual as a social entity, a biological creature, and a spiritual being. Despite the complexity of these issues, I will make an effort to delineate the problem using these three basic divisions.

The Call of Data: Evidence-based Therapy

Part of the conundrum of this exchange is finding a common basis for discussion. Loretta Kopelman has clearly outlined the difficulty of finding adequate definitions to differentiate conventional and alternative medicines, and by implication she accepts that each system occupies some terrain of common ground in the social world of health care and that we must proceed as best we can to compare them. This seems perfectly appropriate to me since, as discussed below, I am distrustful of drawing boundaries too rigidly. Independent of the particulars of the discussion engaged here, certain underlying precepts frame any comparison of health care systems. Disease and human suffering cannot be understood solely from one perspective. The experience of being sick and caring for the ill are different. There are multiple systems of meaning that confer significance and an ordering to such experience. Biomedicine, for all of its explanatory power and therapeutic triumphs, is, finally, an approach to care in constant evolution as it seeks to optimize its own methods and successes. Once those rather self-evident and modest admissions are made, then perhaps we might begin to discern possible links between contesting orientations.

To pursue this point, consider the following schematized version of health care. The ABCs of care fall into a developmental pattern, one in which we might easily regard CAM therapies on a continuum with "conventional" ones. The developmental pattern is "C" (controversial), followed by "B" (clearly best or beneficial), followed by "A" (atavistic) as new therapies evolve. Let us begin with the last. Discarded therapies are regarded as atavistic or archaic. They were regarded as useful and appropriate at one point but now are seen as ineffectual. But such therapies may still be indulged in either out of ignorance or bias. For instance, I might treat a patient with a drug recently shown to be either ineffective or deleterious, or that was simply superseded by a better drug. My use of the older medication reflects my ignorance of the latest data or perhaps a bias against it. The point is, simply, that many patients of conventional practitioners suffer the application of outmoded (and even useless) therapies for one reason or another. These matters are ultimately decided through comparative studies, education, and peer pressure under the guise of practice standards.

The "B" component of clinical care refers to beneficial care. This category reflects the conventional wisdom of the medical community and refers to that body of uncontested therapy, such as iron supplements for iron deficiency anemia or antimicrobials for urinary tract infections. Failure to prescribe such medications for diagnosed ailments would constitute malpractice. By definition, "alternative" therapy falls outside the "B" category. If it were otherwise, there would be no controversy, which introduces the most immediate line of combat, the "C" category.

The "C" therapies are the controversial ones, those conventional *and* CAM therapies that remain outside broad acceptance because no consensus exists as to how a particular disease should be treated. Even within orthodox practice, all too often data for a given therapy are ambiguous or even nonexistent. There is simply too much ignorance or latitude for interpretation to discern the "best" approach. CAM therapists deserve the same process of judgment, but as Tom Whitmarsh laments (and documents), we have a dire paucity of studies to examine even well-demarcated clinical syndromes such as migraine.

Part of the problem of a fair adjudication is that, in more instances than not, the design of the clinical study is not up to proper scientific standards, reflecting the inexperience of the practitioners. Here we come face to face with the chicken-and-egg imbroglio of assessing CAM therapies—how do we enlist those most capable of conducting rigorous clinical studies? If one decides, a priori, that acupuncture, for instance, is placebo at best because the basis of its effects seems preposterous from biomedicine's perspective, then such alternative care is placed in the atavistic category out of hand. But if, as Howard Brody argues, when one examines the data more sympathetically (i.e., assesses efficacy as opposed to consistency with present scientific theory) and concludes that the acupuncturist is achieving therapeutic effects, then acupuncture is moved from an archaic therapy to a controversial one. And, indeed, there is disagreement among medical doctors as to the efficacy of acupuncture.

But this is not the place to argue this example, or any other. More saliently, I wish to move beyond the particulars and make the general claim that the dispute lies at a deeper level than the simple evaluation of the data. As Paul Root Wolpe observes, the truth claims made by each group are radically different when seen within the context of their encompassing belief systems. I maintain that this is the level of real confrontation and will return to this matter later.

Here, I will make a simple assertion built upon the ABC structure: if one appreciates the dynamics of biomedicine's own evolution, then I think it obvious that the position of boundaries between conventional and CAM therapies is ever-changing and therefore difficult to pin down. What is "alternative" at one time might well become "conventional" at another. What some take as wild inference may be a question for another of considered judgment and justifiable interpretation. Medicine is not a formal science and intuition plays a role more prominent than we might like, and physicians often must practice the "art of medicine" with a lack of authoritative scientific knowledge that plagues nonconventional therapies. Be that as it may, a steady stream of so-called alternative approaches enters the medical canon, and one must be wary of dogmatism or predetermined negative prejudice—considering how much of biomedicine itself depends on the ethos of progress and entertainment of fresh ideas. Succinctly stated, it is inappropriate simply to dismiss CAM out of hand, and I suggest that we instead place the discussion of alternative therapies in the "C" category of controversy. And here the call for data is sorely felt.

Despite the National Institutes of Health mandate to explore alternative therapies in a serious and systematic fashion (with a budget of nearly $70 million in 2000),[2] the problem is daunting. Not only is there dispute about the character of such studies (considering the difficulty of defining psychosocial factors), it is vexatious to prioritize among the competing alternative systems being actively pursued by the public. When one considers the state of evidence-based conventional medicine, it is easy to understand the laments of those who see the attention to acupuncture or homeopathy as misplaced as compared to expenditures to assess more "rational" approaches.

But the case for measuring the effects of CAM remains compelling. We must peer, as Janus, simultaneously in two directions. On the one hand, alternative medicine challenges orthodox medicine to examine its own assumptions, its methods of evaluation, its outcomes, and its truth claims. A crucial element of biomedicine is its own critical self-evaluation and scrutiny of its bona fide claims—exactly the same judgments orthodox medicine claims to place before its contenders. This is where David Hufford's critique of Marcia Angell and her fellow travelers is so compelling. The out-of-hand dismissal of claims simply because they do not appear consistent with current dogma is myopic in the extreme. Such a "know-nothing" position seems to me untenable, both practically and philosophically, as Hufford cogently details.

On the other hand, orthodox medicine appropriately demands some measure to assess alternative approaches. While open to anomalies and unknown or unexplained effects, alternative medicine must abide by some judicious assessment. That being said, as Bonnie O'Connor and others argue, the criteria of judgment may need to be broadened in scope to deal more adequately with social and psychological factors. The exercise must be beneficial and useful to society if for no other reason than that orthodox medicine will be strengthened in its self-examination and alternative medicine will either attain or lose its legitimacy beyond simple folk belief. Even if alternative therapies prove to be placebo effects, this does not in itself exclude their efficacy. Ultimately, given the limits of knowledge, we must be satisfied with efficacy and aspire to growing veracity.

Again, hardly anyone would contest the legitimacy of establishing bona fide criteria of care, and the demand for clinical trials of CAM therapies resides in this domain. While I see no realistic alternative, it is important to understand that data alone may not settle the various claims made by nonconventionalists in any final sense, for the contention arises at a deeper level, namely on contested foundations or criteria for assessment. If knowledge is legislated by a particular form of discourse, other rationalities may be either ignored or, when translated, may appear unintelligible. Our only choice is to go forward, but it seems clear that only certain kinds of questions will be addressed, leaving others to be resolved in different ways. Controlled clinical trials are mandatory, but they will fail to address the basic issue: the legitimacy of belief systems seemingly incompatible with Western biomedicine.

CAM and the Legitimacy of the Placebo

Medicine's ancient and still primary calling is the care of the ill. Western societies have endorsed and followed the practice developing from a scientific model of disease, in which a reductive strategy has been employed to dissect the body in molecular and genetic terms.

Having a rational scientific basis, patients who endorse such approaches to their illness enlist the diagnostic and therapeutic tools that have been acquired as products of this belief system. The efficacy of such an approach is undoubtedly effective for certain diseases, but not for all. A host of chronic ailments, nuisance conditions, and psychologically oriented problems have thus far proved resistant to effective therapies from this scientific orientation. For an impatient public whose medical ailments persist in the orthodox setting, other kinds of therapies beckon effectively.

One response on the part of the conventional medical establishment has been the strategic decision to capture these patients because of their economic significance. Paul Root Wolpe notes, correctly I think, that academic departments of medicine have been slow to embrace the challenge of alternative therapies and that the primary impetus for hospitals to offer such services has arisen from those watching the financial ledger. They see lost revenues, and under the rationale of "If we don't get them, others will," various marketing ploys have been instituted to capture those who have wandered astray. The academic medical centers embrace this option under the moral mandate of care. Even if only placebo effects are offered, the ethics of "comprehensive" care affords the justification for opening CAM clinics. If such therapies are offered in a setting where one might assess that no harm is being done—either by commission or omission—then the public is well served.

Placebos are gaining legitimacy in the popular press, not only for the interesting scientific questions they pose but because placebo is also being understood as "effective without scientific explanation." This is the wedge required by those discarding conventional medicine who need a rationale for adopting courses of action other than those prescribed by orthodoxy. The public has been alerted that much of what passes for conventional therapy is placebo. The syllogism being invoked is a simple one: placebos work, we do not know how, but if scientific medicine is also contaminated with "bogus" therapies, who is in a position to judge patient satisfaction more reliably than the patient herself? Howard Brody has taken pains to demonstrate the distortion of such a position, but his insights, which would help frame discussion of this difficult topic, are not acknowledged by all critics.

The opening of the academic center to CAM is seen by many as allowing the fox into the chicken coop. Consider a recent diatribe by Norman Levitt, whose *Prometheus Bedeviled* is an impassioned defense of science.[3] When considering contemporary medicine, the rhetoric becomes almost hysterical. Levitt asserts that scientific medicine is under siege by proponents of CAM. Never mind that he does not (and probably cannot) define "alternative medicine." He sees the ascendancy of public support for clinical nonorthodoxy not only as a sign of science in retreat but also as an alarming public health menace. The "argument" is tortured, but it goes like this: charlatans, like Deepak Chopra, are selling the public a bill of goods that is a mixture of religious and folk beliefs, with some pseudoscientific buzz words, so that the gullible seek in such approaches a reconstitution of their spiritual and material selves. Sidestepping the reasonable allure of such a goal, Levitt again ignores the complexity of the issues he is raising—the nature of healing as both a physiological and psychological/cultural process—and places illness solely within the province of scientific medicine. He sees this as an (exaggerated) opportunity for the forces of antiscience to gain momentum and sweep aside the standing of conventional medicine. Simply denying the legitimacy of such practices is hardly consistent with the openmindedness supposedly characteristic of the scientific mentality.

But putting that matter to the side, Levitt goes on to the second stage of his analysis of medicine by reviewing its sociopolitical history in America, specifically the politico-economic structure of medicine's ruling elite, the recent loss of public trust, the "black box" character of the clinician's technical tools, and seeing in all of these factors elements that conspire and aggregate to work against the scientific ethos of medical practice. The public's awareness of scientific uncertainty is coupled to these forces to undermine the legitimacy of the scientific approach. Levitt regards all of this as playing out some basic irrationality. Here the structure of his thought is revealed: one focused on combating what he perceives as a deeply embedded counterforce to science, not because of any weakness in the philosophical strength of the scientific outlook but rather because he would "acknowledge that some law of intellectual entropy may be a given of the human condition."[4] Medicine is in particular danger because times of pain and fear of death "seem to call forth aspects of our mental proclivities that work at cross-purposes to logical and systematic thought."[5] This is but the most dramatic consequence of our intrinsic irrational, antiscientific characters. On this view, science is indeed precious and precariously holding the forces of darkness at bay.

Accordingly, critics in Levitt's camp argue that medicine in the twenty-first century aspires to a scientific ideal, and therapy must thus be determined by strict criteria of efficacy. If the data are not available (category C, above) then we rather err to the side of conventional approaches, if for no other reason than ideology. Why accept any therapy that arises from a system of thought so alien to our own and of no proven efficacy or veracity? On what basis does a patient determine the course of professional action? Where is the line drawn between patient satisfaction and honest brokering? After a century of a certain model of disease and intervention, why should the fundamental legitimacy of that approach be so easily overturned? If not by our rational standards, by what criteria should we act?

Trained in this tradition, I find it difficult to counter the arguments in these questions as posed. Indeed, I personally do not pursue CAM therapies, and so my response is intellectual, based on philosophical and historical considerations, which I hope can shed some light on the nature of the issues that these plaintive questions address. For me, the "answer" does not lie in testing therapy X or Y (advocates will never be convinced by testers alien to their own tradition) but rather in understanding that reductive-oriented medicine, by its very character, cannot address certain metaphysical issues of the ill. The orthodox versus alternative controversy is not really about which therapy is better but rather which philosophy is better attuned to address the ill. Or perhaps, rather than making an either/or decision, might we better accommodate complementary belief systems to offer patients more comprehensive care or, at least, to accommodate their perceived needs better? Ultimately, this is the question that must be answered.

Historical Perspective

This last question arises from the particular historical development of Western medicine as it became a product of the scientific ethos of the mid-nineteenth century. At that time, two philosophies of science—positivism and reductionism—emerged that decisively shifted the character of medicine toward a new scientific ideal. Neither was a totally novel philosophical strategy—indeed each has a venerable history dating to at least the early modern period—but by the 1850s they were articulated within a new context and were joined to set a new agenda for clinical medicine.

By the end of the century, medical training had been transformed, and application of a laboratory-based approach to therapeutics established revolutionary aspirations for medical practice. The impact of this new objective attitude had a profound influence on the doctor-patient relationship and, even more importantly, gave new meaning to illness and the body. The holistic construct of Man and the medicine that served him were replaced by a fragmenting clinical science that in its powerful ability to dissect the body into its molecular components failed to address the person qua person. In other words, the laboratory context replaced the integrity of the individual with a different standard of fragmenting analysis.

The repercussions of this movement away from a holistic approach to one that celebrated the reductive scrutiny left medicine with a deep contradiction. Initially designed to address the patient's illness as experienced in an array of meanings directly accessible to the sufferer, disease of a system or organ became the focus of concern, and medicine thereby made a Faustian pact with valueless science. Amending, and oftentimes forgoing, integrated care—one that addressed the psychological and spiritual dimensions of illness as well as the pathophysiological—medicine too often was accused of losing its deepest commitment to the patient. Alternative medicine appeals to this deep, metaphysical yearning for wholeness, and, in this sense, the crisis biomedicine is facing (namely, the challenges posed by alternative therapies) represents an accounting for its neglect of this broader human need. Let us delve a bit into the historical and philosophical roots of this issue.

Positivism

For the past century and a half, mainstream science has assumed a positivist stance, one that increasingly seeks to describe the world in nonpersonal terms.[6] Positivism carries several meanings and has been notoriously difficult to define, yet certain precepts may be identified, especially as espoused in its nineteenth-century format. Foremost, it championed a new form of objectivity, one that radically removed the personal report in favor of one that was universally accessible. To be "true" and "real," knowledge had to be attested to by a community of observers who shared common observation. This move from the private sphere of experience to a communal one had begun at the dawn of modern science, but in the mid-nineteenth century the ideal of truth became clearly enunciated as a scientific principle.[7] Thus, positivism sought a collection of rules and evaluative criteria by which to distinguish true knowledge from what Wittgenstein famously called "nonsense," a normative attitude that would regulate how we use such terms as *knowledge, science, cognition,* and *information.*

As developed in the 1850s, positivism came to be understood as a philosophical belief that held that the methods of natural science offer the only viable way of thinking correctly about human affairs. Accordingly, empirical experience—processed with a self-conscious fear of subjective contamination—served as the basis of all knowledge. Facts, the products of sensory experience, and, by extrapolation, the data derived from machines and instruments built as extensions of that faculty, were first ascertained and then classified. "Hypothesis" was defined as the expectation of observing facts of a certain kind under certain conditions, and a scientific "law" could be defined as the proposition that, under certain conditions, facts of a certain kind were uniformly observable. Any hypothesis or law that could not be defined in terms such as these would be written off as "pseudo-hypothesis" or "pseudo-law."

Positivism contrasted with, indeed was constructed in opposition to, the romantic view of the world by denying any cognitive worth to subjective value judgments. Experience, positivists maintained, contains no such qualities of men or events as "noble," "good," "evil," or "beautiful." In radical reaction against the romantics, positivists sought instead to objectify nature, banishing human prejudice from scientific judgment. The total separation of observer from the object of observation—an epistemological ideal—reinforced the positivist disavowal of "value" as part of the process of observation. One might interpret, but such evaluative judgments had no scientific (i.e., objective) standing. Simply put, where the romantics privileged human interpretation (exemplified by artistic imagination), the positivists championed mechanical objectivity (e.g., thermometer, voltmeter, and chemical analysis).[8]

The radical separation of the observing/knowing subject and his object of scrutiny is the single most important characteristic of positivist epistemology. Because of this understanding, positivists claimed that science should rest on a foundation of neutral and dispassionate observation. The more careful the design of the experimental conditions, the more precise the characterization of phenomena, the more likely the diminution of subjective contaminants. Thus the strict positivist confined himself to phenomena and their ascertainable relationships through a vigorous mechanical objectivity. Most pertinent to our interest here, in the life sciences, positivism exercised new standards in the study of physiology that applied the objective methodologies of chemistry and physics to organic processes. This approach allowed newly adopted laboratory techniques to establish physiology as a new discipline and gave birth to biochemistry, whose central tenets held that the fundamental principles of organic and inorganic chemistries were identical, differing only inasmuch as the molecular constituents of living organisms were governed by complex constraints of metabolism.

Reductionism

Positivism's methodology was intimately linked to the assumption that all of nature was of one piece, and the study of life was potentially no different in kind than the study of chemical reactions, the movement of heavenly bodies, or the evolution of mountains. Thus, if all of nature was unified—constituted of the same elements and governed by the same fundamental laws—then the organic world was simply on a continuum with the inorganic. According to this set of beliefs, there was no essential difference between animate and inanimate physics and chemistry, and the organic world was therefore subject to the same kinds of study so successfully applied in physics. Medicine was to treat the body essentially as a machine, governed by uniform chemistry, and thus susceptible to mechanical repair. The new problem was both to reduce the organic to the inorganic, that is, to exhibit the continuity of substance and operation, and concomitantly to understand the distinct character of life processes. To accomplish this twofold agenda, positivism was soon coupled to another philosophy, reductionism.

The reductionists were initially a group of German physiologists, led by Hermann Helmholtz, who in the 1840s openly declared their manifesto of scientific inquiry.[9] They did not argue that certain organic phenomena were not unique, only that all causes must have certain elements in common. They connected biology and physics by equating the ultimate basis of the respective explanations. Reductionism, specifically physical reductionism as opposed to the later development of genetic reductionism, was also a reaction to romanticism's lingering attachment to vitalism, that notion that life possessed a special "life force." Vitalism was attacked because it belied the unity of nature offered by various mechanistic philosophies.

The debate was largely resolved by three key discoveries: Helmholtz's demonstration that heat generated by contracting muscle could be accounted for by chemical metabolism (1847) (that is, no special vitalistic force was necessary); Louis Pasteur showing, about a decade later, that bacteria could not arise through spontaneous (that is, vitalistic) generation; and finally Darwin, who in the *Origin of Species* (1859) presented the case for a blind materialism to explain the evolution of species. The appeal of vitalism was not totally extinguished by mid-century, but certainly a new scientific ethos had taken over the life sciences by 1890. And medicine was radically changed as a result of these developments. In the United States the establishment of the first research-based medical school, Johns Hopkins, the subordination of contenders to biomedicine through the Flexner Report (1910), and the enthusiastic application and still unrealized expectations for the elimination of infectious diseases each date to this period.

Kenneth Schaffner clearly discusses how philosophy of science is now grappling with a fundamental anxiety concerning the "unity of science," where the original aspirations of the reductionists are being modified by the increasingly "local" character of scientific knowledge. If the natural world is seamless, then presumably our scientific approach to its study should also be unified, both epistemologically and metaphysically. But there is growing evidence that the various scientific approaches applied by the different kinds of scientific inquiry are not easily linked to each other to offer a coherent and seamlessly unified picture of the world.[10] Glaring rhetorical and cognitive gaps have been highlighted by historians and sociologists of science, who have claimed that the context of discovery is a critical parameter for truth claims.

Both the pluralism of methodologies and the diverse questions posed by different kinds of study point to the inevitability of disunity, which beyond fragmentary knowledge reflects the relative isolation of highly specialized sciences pursuing their own highly specific agendas with their own highly evolved (and therefore peculiar) methodologies. While science continues to pursue a comprehensive and coherent world view, these critics argue that it is not at all certain that the various strands of scientific pursuit will be unified in any fundamental sense. So, from this critical perspective, it remains highly problematic in defining the basic elements whether parts will effectively be put back together as integrated wholes.

While the debate concerning the eventual success or failure of the reductive program continues, almost all concur that, regardless of current reductive strategies and their accompanying aspirations, more comprehensive modes of organizing and resynthesizing complex systems are required to understand complex physiological function. This conclusion may be drawn as we appreciate the limitations of simple cause and effect relations as defined by linear mechanical models. We are in the infancy of utilizing complexity and chaos theories to address the limits of models developed three centuries ago, but, notwithstanding the applications of these newer orientations or others that will inevitably develop, I believe there is a deeper issue at hand, one perhaps best summarized by William James in 1902:

[Nature] is a vast *plenum* in which our attention draws capricious lines in innumerable directions. We count and name whatever lies upon the special lines we trace, whilst the other things and the untraced lines are neither named nor counted. There are in reality infinitely more things 'unadapted' to each other in this world than there are things 'adapted'; infinitely more things with irregular relations than with regular relations between them. But we look for the regular kind of thing exclusively, and ingeniously discover and preserve it in our memory. It accumulates with other regular kinds, until the collection of them fills our encyclopedias. Yet all the while between and around them lies an infinite anonymous chaos of objects that no one ever thought of together, of relations that never yet attracted our attention.[11]

If this "selection" argument is applied to medicine, we see how, if we cast our conceptual net wide enough, CAM may be regarded as another instance of legitimate study/practice. Operating in a different therapeutic context, truth claims may be fairly championed on the basis of cultural diversity (David Hufford), folk belief/psychology (Bonnie O'Connor), spiritual values (David Larson), and the instability of communal standards for objectivity (Paul Root Wolpe). Thus, advocates of CAM argue that final adjudication about CAM claims must reside in the efficacy of response. Different standards of testing might be applied by different kinds of practitioners (Loretta Kopelman), and if we can somehow find some underlying unity among various approaches, it must be found not in some future "scientific" understanding but in a pragmatic assessment, now (Howard Brody). Each of these discussants argues, explicitly or implicitly, that the verdict of care must occur at the practical level of deciding "what works best." Accordingly, stepping outside current positivist/reductionist boundaries may be required to answer certain clinical questions.

The Quest for Holism

Medicine, of course, was never monolithic, and well into our own century renewed challenges to reductive orthodoxy have appeared, even within mainstream conventional medicine: constitutionalism, psychosomatic medicine, neo-Hippocratic medicine, neo-humoralism, social medicine, Catholic humanism, and, in Europe, homeopathy and naturopathy.[12] These "holistic" systems not only have been espoused by various kinds of practitioners, but, in noteworthy instances, they have been championed by "legitimate" basic scientists—for example, Henry Head,[13] Walter B. Cannon,[14] and Alexandre Besredka.[15] Through historical reflection, we can see that the discussions of today are directly linked to similar debates held between 1920 and 1950, which in turn were reframed arguments dating back to the nineteenth century.

The term "holism" was coined by Jan Smuts in a 1926 bio-philosophical text entitled *Evolution and Holism*.[16] When applied to medicine, holism refers not only to the relational character of medical description and therapy but to the scope of the medical gaze. And more deeply, holism "has not only been about the object of knowledge but about the nature of knowledge,"[17] specifically the requirement for seeking a synthesis of increasingly fragmented knowledge to understand the character of integrated wholes.

This was both an epistemological project and a moral one: the ethical imperative to maintain human relations always marked holism in opposition to the underlying positivist orientation that sought to minimize the human element.[18] The conflict rightly has been seen as an extension of deeper cultural conflicts, and in some contexts, such as in France and Germany, the polemics extended quite clearly into the broadest of political and philosophical ideologies. This is hardly the place to pursue this aspect of the holism/reductionism debate other than to note its broad application beyond medicine proper, suggesting that the cultural forces at play in the specific medical setting are composed, at least in part, from contributing elements arising from other social and intellectual agendas. So while the holist rejoinder of the interwar years has been well studied, it is perhaps less evident how our own era may be showing similar protestations and unease with the conditions of contemporary life that are reflected in the current espousal of alternative therapies.

Another critical caveat about the reductive-holistic balance is each position's unsteady configuration with the other. As Charles Rosenberg has observed, holism is ultimately defined in contrast to, and in the context of, the prevailing reductionism of the era: holism and reductionism are inexorably coupled and cannot be defined independent of each other.[19] He further opines that, in general, holism's plea is not against reductive explanation but a warning against premature and unsophisticated reductionism, where the limits of a reductionist approach are either unknown or unacknowledged.

These points are quite germane to this discussion, for I believe that the doctor-patient encounter is by its very nature a negotiated attempt to coordinate, if not combine, different frames of reference. In treating disease, medical science employs a reductive approach, while the patient experiencing illness assumes a holistic stance. Each has its place and each must accommodate the other. So it seems to me that the recurrent question plaguing a reductionist, positivistic clinical medicine is to what extent the mechanistic, dehumanizing experience of becoming a medical object of scrutiny and therapy can be mitigated by counterbalancing factors. I have argued elsewhere for the primacy of the humane calling, subordinating science and technology to the broader ethical imperative.[20] Here I would only suggest that if contemporary orthodox medical care is facing a crisis in public confidence, then the answer lies in its failure to address the humane needs of its patients. How to reestablish a stable balance of reductive science and holistic care must dominate the agenda of proving or disproving the efficacy of alternative approaches. Ultimately, clinical science will "win" only if it can effectively deal with the same humane issues CAM currently often addresses more effectively.

In short, if we pragmatically move beyond the dispute about relativism (which is really an argument about the dominance of one world view over another), then the discussion begins where my comments were initiated, namely, that there is a sociological question that must be answered: why do so many people flock to CAM? The trivial answer to this filtered question is that, presumably, their respective illnesses/discomforts/maladjustments are more effectively addressed in these alternative settings. The significant question is *why?* Underlying each chapter of this volume lurks this question, and the various "answers" offered refract the problem in different ways and thus arrive at various "solutions." In their composite we witness not only the fragmented character of how we regard the question but the obvious complexity of formulating a comprehensive response.

I have taken some pains to place the discussion framing this collection of essays within a particular philosophical and historical context because I see the discussion as pointing back to a historical period when a turn in the road was made, when the path of holism was sidetracked to make room for a strategy of reification that left issues of integration subordinate to the technical mastery of disease. Despite the extraordinary power of this new approach and its undeniable success, we are facing a crisis of public dissatisfaction. The debate about CAM, however, is not "simply" about medicine but spills over into a deep conflict about differing world views. To initiate debate, CAM advocates demand acknowledgment of the plurality of science and the necessary limits of scientific medicine. This may well be the most contentious and single greatest obstacle to effective debate about alternative medicine because the issues are so firmly embedded in beliefs inaccessible to open discussion.

Because differing metaphysics generally remain intractable to resolution, I regard any accommodation to CAM from the biomedical perspective as following two courses already established within scientific interest. The first is continuing study of the placebo. Howard Brody makes the cogent point that the placebo response minimizes the difference between conventional and alternative medicines, and in appreciating the placebo effect we are alerted to the difficulty of teasing out the various silent factors of natural disease, psychosocial influences, and "hidden" physiologies. But obtaining data in even the best-intended of studies cannot necessarily decide the matter in dispute. The placebo is probably our best bridge concept for linking scientific medicine with its contenders, but the very notion of "placebo" is itself poorly understood, representing an array of unknowns. It demands even more careful scrutiny than we already afford to that proportion of patients whose diseases evolve from one state of illness to another. Perhaps one of the most important contributions alternative medicine will make to orthodoxy is the renewed demand on the part of conventional methodologies to find the means for assessing clinical outcomes, in whatever setting.

The second conduit for study of CAM is the randomized clinical trial (RCT), the gold standard of clinical evaluation for the past fifty years. But the RCT itself is facing new challenges, beyond the obvious needs of appropriate application to assess CAM therapies, an issue well discussed by Asbjørn Hróbjartsson and Stig Brorson. We have long realized that RCTs can only give us relative, not absolute, responses, but as Wayne Jonas shows, the complexity of assessing alternative therapies demands that we review and revise the RCT to include factors that may not be adequately assessed by current methods. Kenneth Schaffner thus argues that "what works" incorporates two core senses of causation—an efficient cause (typical mechanical cause/effect relationships), where manipulation or intervention initiates effects we can measure, and a final cause, which incorporates the notion of a "required" way. This second modality refers to the need of the assessment to follow conventional understanding of cause/effect relationships, which in the medical setting may not always be possible to apply, for patient participation or community development often appear as a crucial element in the therapeutic intervention. In such cases, the RCT cannot be employed effectively, and its role as final adjudicator is undermined. In other words, the positivist ideal is not always applicable.

I do not see the limits of the RCT as a manifestation of the disunity of science so much as the disunity of experience. "Science" has a circumscribed domain whose boundaries, as changing and elusive as they might be, must be acknowledged. And it is here at this definitional ambiguity that the character of medicine becomes more fully portrayed, breaking through its enclosure within the walls of the laboratory. While I see the arbitrating role of the RCT and better appreciation of the placebo, these paths of inquiry seek to bring CAM into the biomedical fold. I doubt that such a strategy will quell the revolt, for the crisis facing orthodox medicine is over a deeper issue, namely a struggle of defining medicine. In accepting that medicine is a science, it well behooves us also to acknowledge that the traditional aspirations of science are simply inadequate to address medicine's moral mission of care. Care encompasses more than understanding genes, proteins, and organs; it also must address the needs of the psyche and the person embedded in culture. Compromising the deep commitment to comprehensive care in the name of "science" is to forfeit medicine's ultimate responsibility, which is not toward the establishment of its scientific character but rather toward its mandate to care for the patient.

Alternative care providers have reminded physicians of the principal commitments to the ill and the basis of public confidence. Authority resides not only in knowledge but in the trust engendered by compassion. These are lessons that arise outside the boundaries of science and clearly mark those limits. Even if the challenge of CAM offers no new therapies, it has, at the very least, forced the American public to reassess the character of our medicine and consider the need for substantive examination of assumptions that have been firmly in place for over a century. To those decrying the mode or origin of this critique, I would only note that CAM's own approach need not be "correct," it must only be effective in nudging our complacency into more creative pathways of self-examination. My own faith in science's power and its humane application motivates me in welcoming all honest brokers into dialogue. For those seeking a well-balanced representation of that discussion, this collection is a superb place to listen.

NOTES

1. David M. Eisenberg et al., "Unconventional Medicine in the United States. Prevalence, Costs, and Patterns of Use," *NEJM* 328, no. 4 (1993): 246–52.

2. Erik Stokstad, "Stephen Straus's Impossible Job," *Science* 288, no. 5471 (2000): 1568–70.

3. Norman Levitt, *Prometheus Bedeviled: Science and the Contradictions of Contemporary Culture* (New Brunswick, N.J.: Rutgers University Press, 1999).

4. Levitt, *Prometheus Bedeviled*, p. 206.

5. Levitt, *Prometheus Bedeviled*, p. 209.

6. Walter M. Simon, *European Positivism in the Nineteenth Century* (Ithaca, N.Y.: Cornell University Press, 1963).

7. Leszek Kolakowski, *The Alienation of Reason: A History of Positivist Thought,* translated by Norbert Guterman (Garden City, N.J.: Doubleday, 1968).

8. Lorraine Daston, "Wordless Objectivity," in *Little Tools of Knowledge: Historical Essays on Academic and Bureaucratic Practice,* ed. P. Becker and W. Clark (Ann Arbor: University of Michigan Press, 2000).

9. David H. Galaty, "The Philosophical Basis for Mid-nineteenth Century German Reductionism," *Journal of the History of Medicine and Allied Sciences* 29 (1974): 295–316.

10. Peter Galison and David J. Stump, eds., *The Disunity of Science: Boundaries, Contexts, and Power* (Stanford: Stanford University Press, 1996).

11. William James, *The Varieties of Religious Experience* (New York: The Library of America, 1987), p. 394.

12. Christopher Lawrence and George Weisz, "Medical Holism: The Context" in *Greater than the Parts: Holism in Biomedicine 1920–1950,* ed. Christopher Lawrence and George Weisz (Oxford and New York: Oxford University Press, 1998), pp. 1–22.

13. L. S. Jacyna, "Questions of Identity: Science, Aesthetics, and Henry's Head," in *Greater than the Parts,* pp. 211–33.

14. Allan Young, "Walter Cannon and the Psychophysiology of Fear," in *Greater than the Parts,* pp. 234–56.

15. Ilana Lowy, " 'The Terrain Is All': Metchnikoff's Heritage at the Pasteur Institute, from Besredka's 'Antivirus' to Bardach's 'Orthobiotic Serum,' " in *Greater than the Parts,* pp. 257–82.

16. Jan C. Smuts, *Holism and Evolution* (New York: Macmillan, 1926).

17. Lawrence and Weisz, "Medical Holism," p. 3.

18. H. Stuart Hughes, *Consciousness and Society: The Reorientation of European Social Thought, 1890–1930* (Frogmore, St. Albans, United Kingdom: Paladin, 1974).

19. Charles Rosenberg, "Holism in Twentieth-century Medicine," in *Greater than the Parts,* pp. 335–55.

20. Alfred I. Tauber, *Confessions of a Medicine Man: An Essay in Popular Philosophy* (Cambridge, Mass.: MIT Press, 1999).

Contributors

HOWARD BRODY received an M.D. and a Ph.D. in philosophy from Michigan State University and completed his family practice residency at the University of Virginia. He has been on the faculty of Michigan State University since 1980 and from 1985 to 2000 was director of the Center for Ethics and Humanities in the Life Sciences. He is particularly interested in the clinical and ethical aspects of the physician-patient relationship in primary care. He wrote *Placebos and the Philosophy of Medicine: Clinical, Conceptual, and Ethical Issues* (University of Chicago Press, 1980), *Stories of Sickness* (Yale University Press, 1987), and *The Healer's Power* (Yale University Press, 1992). He recently coauthored (with Daralyn Brody) *The Placebo Response: How You Can Release the Body's Inner Pharmacy for Better Health* (HarperCollins, 2000).

STIG BRORSON is a research assistant in the Department of Medical Philosophy and Clinical Theory at the University of Copenhagen. He has an M.D. from the University of Copenhagen. He has published philosophical works on Ludwik Fleck and Thomas S. Kuhn and contributed to the analysis of the sociocultural preconditions of medical cognition. He is currently involved in research on the philosophical basis of taxonomy and central concepts in medicine.

DANIEL CALLAHAN, a cofounder and former president of The Hastings Center, is now director of its International Program. He is also a senior fellow at Harvard Medical School. He received a B.A. from Yale and a Ph.D. in philosophy from Harvard. He is an elected member of the Institute of Medicine and the National Academy of Sciences, as well as a fellow of the American Association for the Advancement of Science. He is the author or editor of numerous books, most recently *False Hopes: Why America's Quest for Perfect Health Is a Recipe for Failure* (Simon & Schuster, 1998).

ASBJØRN HRÓBJARTSSON is a hospital physician at the Medical Centre at Amager Hospital, University of Copenhagen. He has an M.D. from the University of Copenhagen and an M.Phil. in medical philosophy from Glasgow University. His main professional interests are in clinical research methodology and medical philosophy, especially the concepts of placebo and placebo effect and the role of bias in randomized clinical trials and meta-analyses.

DAVID HUFFORD is professor of medical humanities, with joint appointments in behavioral science and family medicine, at the Penn State College of Medicine, where he is also director of the Doctors Kienle Center for Humanistic Medicine. At the University of Pennsylvania he is adjunct professor of religious studies and a faculty member of the Master in Bioethics Program. Hufford received his B.A. degree from Lycoming College and his M.A. and Ph.D. from the University of Pennsylvania. His teaching and research have centered on medicine and culture, complementary and alternative medicine, and religion, spirituality, and health since he joined the college of medicine faculty in 1974. He is currently completing a book on the role of cross-culturally stable spiritual experiences in the development of widespread patterns of belief.

WAYNE B. JONAS, M.D., is director of the Samueli Institute for Information Biology at the Uniformed Services University of the Health Sciences (USUHS) in Bethesda, Maryland. He is a family physician and a fellow of the American Academy of Family Physicians. Before coming to USUHS he was the director of the National Center for Complementary and Alternative Medicine at the National Institutes of Health (NIH) and the director of the Medical Research Fellowship at the Walter Reed Army Institute of Research. He has served as chair of the Program Advisory Council for the NIH Office of Alternative Medicine and as director of a World Health Organization Collaborating Center for Traditional Medicine, and as a member of the Cochrane Collaboration's Group on the Quality of Controlled Clinical Trials and of field groups on primary care and complementary medicine. Jonas has received training in a variety of complementary therapies including diet and nutritional therapy, homeopathy, mind/body methods, electro-acupuncture diagnostics, and clinical pastoral education. He has authored over sixty publications, including the major textbook *Essentials of Complementary and Alternative Medicine* (Lippincott Williams & Wilkins, 1999).

LORETTA M. KOPELMAN, PH.D., is professor and current and founding chair of the Department of Medical Humanities at The Brody School of Medicine at East Carolina University. She has published over one hundred book chapters and articles. She is a member of the editorial board of the *Journal of Medicine and Philosophy, Medical Humanities*, and of the executive council of the Association for the Advancement of Philosophy and Psychiatry. She served on the editorial board of the *Encyclopedia of Bioethics,* second edition. Her publications reflect her interest in rights and welfare of patients and research subjects, including children and vulnerable populations, death and dying, moral problems in psychiatry, research ethics, and other issues in philosophy of medicine and bioethics. She has edited *The Rights of Children and Retarded Persons* (Rock Point, 1978); *Ethics and Mental Retardation*, with John C. Moskop (D. Reidel, 1984); *Children and Health Care: Moral and Social Issues*, with John C. Moskop (Kluwer, 1989); and *Building Bioethics: Conversations with Clouser and Friends on Medical Ethics* (Kluwer, 1999).

DAVID B. LARSON, M.D., M.S.P.H., is president of the National Institute for Healthcare Research and adjunct professor in the Department of Psychiatry and Behavioral Science at Duke University Medical Center and at Northwestern University Medical Center. He worked for twelve years as a senior research officer in the Office of the Director of the National Institutes of Health, the Office of the Secretary of the Department of Health and Human Services, and the Mental Health Services Branch of the National Institute of Mental Health. He completed his psychiatry residency, chief residency, and geriatric fellowship training at Duke University Medical Center. He received a three-year epidemiology fellowship from the National Institutes of Health during which he earned an M.S.P.H. in epidemiology from the School of Public Health at the University of North Carolina. He has over 240 professional publications, with particular research interests in the influence of spiritual/religious commitment on physical and mental health status and care, the use of systematic reviews in analyzing policy-relevant research, and the provision and delivery of mental health services in both the primary care and specialty mental health sectors. Recent publications include *The Scientific Research on Spirituality and Health: A Consensus Report* (National Institute for Health Care Research, 1998) and *Handbook of Religion and Health* (Oxford University Press, 2001).

SUSAN S. LARSON, M.A.T., is a Phi Beta Kappa graduate of Indiana University in English and comparative literature and earned her master's degree at Duke University. An award-winning journalist and coauthor (with David Larson) of *The Forgotten Factor in Physical and Mental Health: What Does the Research Show?* (National Institute for Healthcare Research, 1994), she has coauthored numerous professional publications and edits *Research Reports* for the National Institute for Healthcare Research.

BONNIE O'CONNOR, PH.D., is a folklorist, ethnographer, and medical educator whose specialty areas include complementary/alternative medicine, cultural issues in health care, and lay people's/patients' experiences of and viewpoints on health, illness, and care. She earned her B.A. in English from Smith College and her master's and doctoral degrees in folklore and folklife at the University of Pennsylvania, where she specialized in the ethnographic study of health belief systems. She has published focused studies of the home birth movement in the United States, the HIV alternative therapies movement, and the meeting of Hmong and biomedical cultural values in a U.S. hospital, as well as more general material in her fields of research and scholarship, including *Healing Traditions: Alternative Medicine and the Health Professions* (University of Pennsylvania Press, 1995). O'Connor is currently codirector and education coordinator of the Brown University Faculty Development in Pediatrics program, Department of Pediatrics of Rhode Island Hospital and the Brown University School of Medicine.

KENNETH F. SCHAFFNER received his M.D. from the University of Pittsburgh and a Ph.D. in philosophy from Columbia University. He is University Professor of Medical Humanities and professor of philosophy at the George Washington University. He has published extensively on alternative research design issues and the ethics of clinical trials and has recently been investigating ethical issues in genetically based research on schizophrenia prevention. He is the author of *Discovery and Explanation in Biology and Medicine* (University of Chicago Press, 1993). He is currently completing a book with the working title "Genes, Development, Behavior and Learning: Conceptual and Methodological Issues."

ALFRED I. TAUBER, M.D., is a professor of medicine and of philosophy, as well as a practicing hematologist and director of the Center for

Philosophy and History of Science at Boston University. He is author of *The Immune Self, Theory or Metaphor?* (Cambridge University Press, 1994), *Confessions of a Medicine Man* (MIT Press, 1999), and *Henry David Thoreau and the Moral Agency of Knowing* (University of California Press, 2001), and coauthor of *Metchnikoff and the Origins of Immunology: From Metaphor to Theory* (Oxford University Press, 1991) and *The Generation of Diversity* (Harvard University Press, 1997). He is editor of several anthologies, including *The Elusive Synthesis: Science and Aesthetics* (Kluwer, 1996) and *Science and the Quest for Reality* (NYU Press, 1997). Author of over one hundred papers concerning the biochemistry of inflammation, he now devotes his primary efforts to nineteenth- and twentieth-century philosophy and history of science and contemporary ethics.

THOMAS E. WHITMARSH, M.D., is a consultant physician at Glasgow Homeopathic Hospital in the Directorate of Medical Specialties within North Glasgow Hospitals NHS Trust, and an honorary clinical lecturer at Glasgow University. He aims to blend the best of orthodox and complementary medical approaches to alleviate the distress of patients, many of whom have chronic and painful conditions that have not been fully addressed by conventional methods. He was a research fellow at the Princess Margaret Migraine Clinic, Charing Cross Hospital, London, and now runs a headache clinic in the Department of Medicine and Therapeutics at the Western Infirmary in Glasgow, where he tries to use as broad a range of therapies as possible to maximize the benefits to headache sufferers. He is on the editorial boards of and contributes regularly to *The British Homeopathic Journal* and *The Journal of Alternative and Complementary Medicine*.

PAUL ROOT WOLPE, PH.D., is a fellow of the Center of Bioethics at the University of Pennsylvania, where he holds faculty appointments in the Department of Psychiatry and the Department of Sociology, and a senior fellow of the university's Leonard Davis Institute of Health Economics. He is chief, Protection of Research Subjects and Patients for the National Aeronautics and Space Administration (NASA). He received his Ph.D. in medical sociology from Yale University. His interests cover a range of topics in sociology, medicine, and bioethics, including the reception of unconventional forms of medical thought by the biomedical establishment in the United States, medical ideology, and the changing health care system. He is the coauthor (with Janell L. Carroll) of the textbook *Sexuality and Gender in Society* (HarperCollins, 1996) and of the forthcoming *Manual for End-of-Life Decision-Making* and has contributed to a variety of encyclopedias on alternative medicine and other bioethical issues.

Index